Heike Höfler

No More Neck Pain!

9-Step Program for Your Neck, Shoulders & Head

Sterling Publishing Co., Inc.

New York

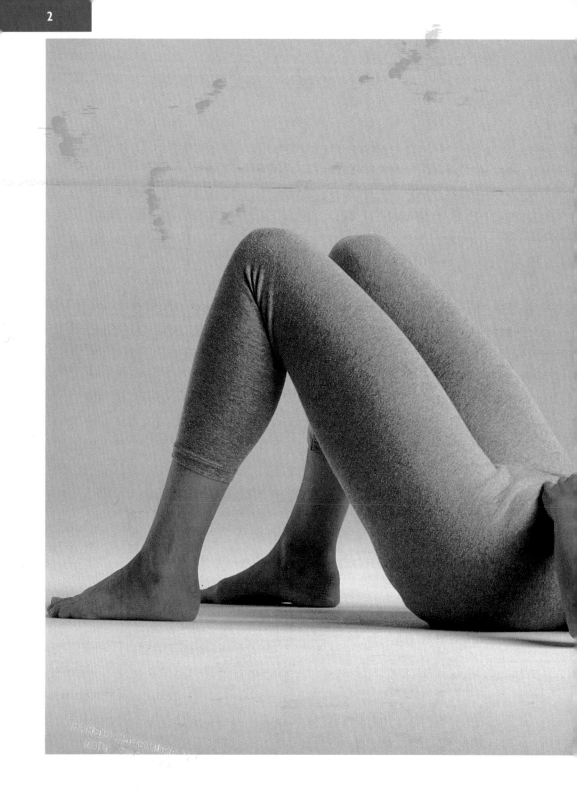

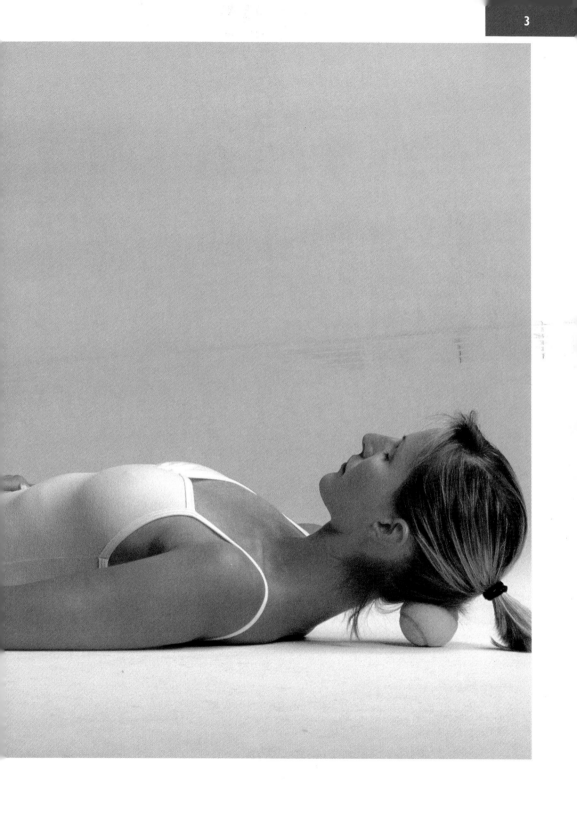

Ɛ⎱ℓ

**Library of Congress Cataloging-in-
Publication Data Available**

Photos: Ulli Seer

10 9 8 7 6 5 4 3 2 1

Published by Sterling Publishing Company, Inc.
387 Park Avenue South,
New York, N.Y. 10016
Originally Published in Germany under the title
Die Nackenschule and © 1998 by BLV
Verlagsgesellschaft GmbH, München
English Translation © 1999 by Sterling Publishing
Co., Inc.
Distributed in Canada by
Sterling Publishing
^{c}/o Canadian Manda Group,
One Atlantic Avenue, Suite 105
Toronto, Ontario
Canada M6K 3E7
Distributed in Great Britain and Europe by
Cassell PLC
Wellington House, 125 Strand
London WC2R 0BB, England
Distributed in Australia by
Capricorn Link (Australia) Pty Ltd.
P.O. Box 6651, Baulkham Hills
Business Centre, NSW 2153,
Australia

Manufactured in the United States of America
Sterling ISBN 0-8069-5937-1

About the author

Heike Höfler, born in 1956, is a certified
sports and gymnastics teacher with many
years of experience. She has been the
director of special courses in back training
and breathing exercises. Höfler has published numerous books with special exercise programs for pregnant women and
for retrogression, breathing, and back
training. She has become widely popular
with fitness training for the face, which
she developed.

Contents

Introduction

We live in an age of inactivity and repetitive motions. This is true for individuals who sit at a desk and for those who work on a computer. But it is equally true for the hair stylist, dentist, electrician, construction worker, supermarket cashier, or the homemaker who is always on the go.

People develop their own peculiar type of posture or movement over the course of their lives. This results in movement patterns that we perform over and over again, subconsciously and automatically.

If these patterns are harmful, over time they result in disorders in the locomotor system and in muscle strains.

Prevention

In recent years, we've noticed a tremendous increase in illnesses and disorders that develop because of the asymmetrical use of the locomotor system. Such symptoms do not occur overnight; they develop almost imperceptibly at first. Then, they become increasingly obvious.

Therefore, the earlier you start a prevention regimen, the easier it is to prevent long-term injury. Preventing the problem produces better results than waiting until you feel the first pains. If you already have pains, you need to restore muscular equilibrium with targeted exercises. These will stretch and relax individual muscle groups and strengthen atrophied parts of the body. Only then will the vertebrae with their joints, ligaments, and disks be preserved, relieved, and cared for.

The importance of body awareness

The first problems begin to develop as early as elementary school. In school, children sit for hours in chairs that are often bad for their posture. In their free time, children often sit too long in front of the television or the computer.

As adults, we face the danger of muscle or joint disorders becoming even more pronounced, leading to serious disorders.

For this reason, exercises alone are not enough. We must also train our bodies so that we can recognize when we assume poor or dangerous posture. We must know how we can preserve the spinal column by not stressing it asymmetrically and by not cramping it.

In recent years, as the personal computer has become increasingly common in offices and businesses, the illnesses and disorders of the cervical vertebral column region have increased tremendously.

Most people who have performed computer or desk work for several years complain about pain in the back of the neck, and not only when they are performing such work.

The sooner we master the economic use of movements, as well as a posture that is friendly to the spinal column at the work station,

the greater the chance of preventing associated illnesses.

Gymnastics is the best medicine

Physicians, especially orthopedists, barely have time today to inform their patients about the gymnastics exercises that are helpful. The physicians themselves often lack expert knowledge in this part of treatment.

Thus, the tips in this book are just as helpful to the health care professional as to the patient; physical therapists, of course, can learn a great deal from it.

Some managed health care programs don't cover courses in prevention, even though prevention is obviously less expensive and more effective than therapy after problems arise. In addition, natural therapy has far fewer side effects than therapy with injections and medications.

As a result of recent cost reductions in health care, many massage therapists have had to close their practices.

However, the complaints about pain in the region of the spinal column, especially in the cervical area, have increased. Therefore, you need to do something before you experience neck problems.

If it's a pain in the neck . . .

The cervical portion of the spinal column is the weakest and most flexible part of the spinal column. This means that it is also the most injury prone.

Emotional problems and mood swings are also felt here. When you are too burdened, stressed, or angry, you automatically tense up in the shoulder and neck region, but, while you're trying to keep a stiff upper lip, your neck becomes stiff as well.

Whenever you tense up, you extend the cervical portion of the spinal column too far forward. If you are sad or depressed, you hold your head down and become too relaxed in this area. There is no longer any healthy tension. The neck muscles are loose and no longer form the necessary muscle corset for the vertebrae. This leads to wear and to disk problems.

Be active for better health

Now, summon the energy and do something for your cervical vertebrae every day! You will find all the important exercises in this book.

Take advantage of any free time during your busy schedule—even if it is only for five minutes—to select two or three exercises and do yourself and your spinal column some good. Get used to scheduling short exercise breaks at your workplace. Use this time for physical activity.

The more frequently and regularly you exercise, the faster you will notice just how good exercise is for you. You'll help your cervical vertebrae, your head (if you suffer from headaches), your concentration, your stamina, and your psyche. Regular exercise strengthens all of you.

Anatomical problem areas around the spinal column

The spinal column

The spinal column consists of thirty-three vertebrae stacked on top of each other like building blocks (Figure 1). Nine of these are fused together to form the sacrum and the coccyx, both of which are inflexible.

The twenty-four flexible vertebrae are divided into five lumbar, twelve thoracic, and seven cervical vertebrae. They are connected to each other by disks, ligaments, muscles, and bony arches.

The spinal column has a double S-curve shape. This enables it to absorb shocks and twists. The S-curve is formed by a lumbar area

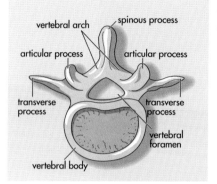

Figure 2
The structure of a vertebra

(concave), a thoracic area (convex), and a cervical area (concave).

A vertebra is composed of the vertebral body, the two vertebral arches that form the vertebral foramen, the two transverse processes,

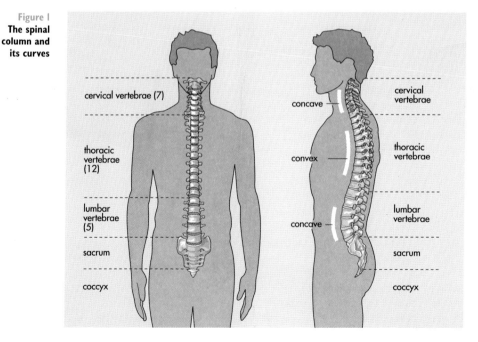

Figure 1
The spinal column and its curves

the two articular processes, and a spinous process that can usually be felt along the back. All of the vertebral foramina together form the spinal canal, which contains and protects the spinal cord and the nerve roots (Figure 2).

The sides of the vertebral arches have notches. Together with the adjacent vertebrae, these form the intervertebral foramina, through which the spinal nerves exit (Figure 3).

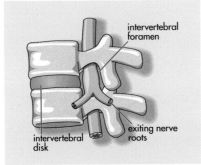

Figure 3
Two vertebrae with the vertebral arch, the spinal cord, and the exiting nerve roots

intervertebral foramen

exiting nerve roots

intervertebral disk

The spinous processes and the transverse processes influence the muscles because they are the sites of action and levers. If the muscles are tense, these processes feel especially painful.

The superior and inferior articular processes together with those of the adjacent vertebrae form a vertebral joint that connects the individual vertebrae in a flexible manner. The joint capsules of the vertebral joints are equipped with many fine nerve endings, including pain fibers. These are the source of much spinal column pain.

The spinal column, also referred to as the central axial organ, supports the head, stabilizes erect posture, permits movement in all directions, and protects the spinal cord. By nature, it is very flexible, but it can lose its flexibility due to age, wear, injury, and poor posture.

The intervertebral disks

An intervertebral disk lies between every two vertebrae, with the exception of the first two cervical vertebrae. The disk acts as a shock absorber for the adjacent vertebral bodies. Healthy intervertebral disks are important for a healthy spinal column.

The bulbous, snugly fitting ring consists of collagen fibers that can retain water and swell up; this swelling action maintains the distance between the vertebral bodies.

In the middle, lies the pulpy nucleus. This has a high water content and declines with age. It distributes weight uniformly on the disk and functions as a ball bearing.

The relationship between metabolism and movement

Local metabolic disturbances are the cause of many injuries to the intervertebral disks. In this context it is important to know:

The intervertebral disks require movement.

These disks contain no blood vessels. They are nourished by diffusion caused by compression and decompression (a pumping and suction mechanism). The longer you sit or stand without moving or changing your posture, the worse this is for the intervertebral disks. Different types of movements are necessary to counter this inaction. These are movements you don't always perform naturally. Thus, targeted exercises are necessary for the welfare of these spinal column parts.

Stress on the intervertebral disks

When you sit or stand all day, the intervertebral disks are barely nourished because there is always pressure on them. Decompressing the disks now and then by leaning against something or by lying down is good for them. Stretching and loosening exercises, as well as tensing and relaxing exercises, are also good.

For example, a posture in which the head is constantly bent forward, the norm in many occupations and in household and leisure activities, is harmful to the cervical disks. This position compresses the disks together forward, while the pulpy nucleus moves out of alignment backward. The situation is similar to a posture in which you hold your head to one side. This posture is fairly common, although people are not usually aware of it.

> **Axiom: Sitting, standing, or stooping perpendicular to the floor produces uniform pressure on the intervertebral disk, and this posture helps the disks buffer the pressure. Incorrect or sloppy posture results in asymmetrical pressure on the disks.**

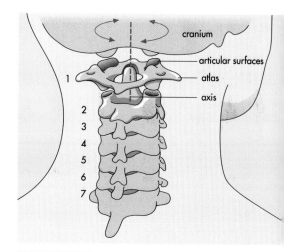

Figure 4
The cervical vertebral column with contrasted first and second cervical vertebrae: Interaction between the occiput (the back of the head), the atlas, and the axis allows the head a wide range of mobility.

The cervical vertebral column

The uppermost section of the spinal column consists of seven vertebrae with their accompanying ligaments, muscles, and joints. This part of the spinal column is the most flexible, a condition that carries risks such as susceptibility to injury and to early wear.

The two uppermost vertebrae, the atlas and the axis, have a different structure than the other cervical vertebrae (Figure 4).

The head joints, which make fine-tuned movements of the head possible, are also unique. No intervertebral disk lies between them. If this were not the case, moving the head would be more cumbersome.

Vertebral arteries pass through the holes in the transverse processes of the cervical vertebrae on both the right and left sides; these arteries supply the brain with fresh oxygen (Figure 5). The spinal cord, with its hundreds of thousands of nerve bundles, runs through the spinal canal. Nerve paths, similar to elec-

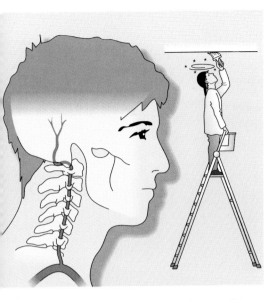

Figure 5
The path of the cervical vertebral artery through the transverse processes of the vertebrae: When you work above your head, you increase the pressure on the artery, impairing the circulation.

trical wires, run from the spinal canal of the cervical vertebral column to the arms and hands. This is why disturbances and poor posture in the cervical vertebral column can affect the arms and hands, producing numbness in the fingers, etc.

Head joints

You can move your head back against the cervical vertebral column by using the two uppermost cervical vertebrae. These join the spinal column to the cranium and bear most of the weight of the head.

The first cervical vertebra, the atlas, is a bony ring without a vertebral body or spinous process. It has two powerful transverse processes that bear the articular surfaces for the joint connections with the cranium and the second cervical vertebra, the axis. Some people can feel these processes below the mastoid process of their temporal bone.

The head rests on the oval artic-ular surfaces, the atlanto-occipital joint. These lie between the head and the uppermost vertebra. Two articular processes, located on the occipital bone, fit perfectly onto the articular surfaces of the atlas. They are somewhat like the rockers of a rocking chair, and together they form a saddle joint. In this joint, the head can rock back and forth about 10∞ without the neck moving also.

The second cervical vertebra possesses a powerful body. At the superior end, there is a toothlike process, the dens axis. This process is the center of movement between the atlas and the axis. It guides the atlas laterally so that when the head turns, the ring of the atlas rotates around the tooth of the axis (Figure 6). Moving the cervical vertebral column is possible in the superior and inferior head joints:

- In the superior head joint between the atlas and occipital bone, the motion occurs in a transverse axis as a nodding movement.
- In the inferior head joint, the atlas rotates with the cranium, which it supports, around the tooth of the axis. This movement makes it possible for you

Figure 6
The atlas and the axis
1. The transverse ligament of the atlas prevents the tooth of the axis from moving toward the spinal cord.
2. Tooth of the axis
3. Anterior arch of the atlas
4. Articular surface between the first and second cervical vertebrae
5. Articular surface between the atlas and the occipital articular process
6. Foramen for the vertebral artery
7. Transverse process of the atlas
8. Posterior arch of the atlas
9. Transverse process of the axis
10. Vertebral body of the axis

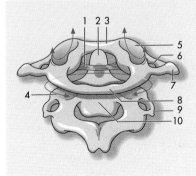

to turn your head around the longitudinal axis.

Bending and extending movements take place in the superior head joint. If the neck remains constantly hyperextended, the articular surfaces will be worn down asymmetrically. The pressure ratios in the vertebral joints change and are no longer optimal.

The spinal cord and the spinal cord nerves

The spinal cord is part of the central nervous system. It is a cable of nerve tissues that becomes part of the elongated cord of the brain at the superior edge of the atlas vertebra in the region of the occipital foramen. Located in the spinal column, the cord is about 17 inches (43cm) long and extends down to the first lumbar vertebra. Thirty-one pairs of spinal cord nerves (spinal nerves) leave the spinal canal laterally through the intervertebral foramina (Figure 7).

The spinal cord has a direct connection to the brain. Think of it as a connecting and switching point for the nerves that enter and exit the spinal cord from certain organs, muscles, and tissues. Nerve impulses to the muscles of the upper extremities (brachial plexus) are sent from the lower cervical part of the spinal cord.

Maintaining an adequate supply of blood to the spinal nerves is important to the structures they control. Thus, the spinal column, which provides protection, can become a problem if it is diseased, if it becomes worn-out or deformed, or if intervertebral disk

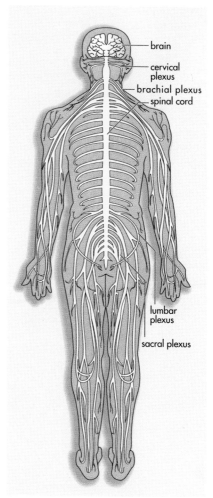

Figure 7
The path of the spinal cord and spinal nerves

brain

cervical plexus

brachial plexus

spinal cord

lumbar plexus

sacral plexus

tissue escapes. Also, overexerted, inflamed, or cramped muscles can press on a nerve and cause pain. A prickling sensation, a feeling of abnormal pressure, and an abnormal temperature perception may result; tingling in the fingers and even symptoms of paralysis occur.

Spinal cord nerves in the cervical vertebral column

Constantly inclining your head to one side (for example, in the case of scoliosis or an asymmetrical

work posture) can lead to degener-
ation and weakening of one or
more intervertebral disks in the
cervical vertebral column. The
pressure compresses the disk on
one side, and the nucleus migrates
to the other or far side.
Intervertebral disk tissue can press
against exiting nerves.

If the disturbance occurs in the
lower cervical area, pain can radiate
out from the shoulder via the arm
to the hand. A sensation of numbness that may actually include
symptoms of paralysis becomes
noticeable in the fingers.
Disturbances in a more anterior
area frequently result in dizziness
and headaches that vary in severity
from mild to migraine.

Arteries of the head and cervical vertebral column

Important arteries to the head trav-
el through the cervical vertebral
column. The blood that flows
through them supplies the brain
with adequate oxygen.

The central nervous system
requires sufficient oxygen and suf-
fers if the blood or oxygen supply
is deficient.

Two pairs of arteries supply the
brain:
• Internal carotid artery (Figure 8)
• Vertebral artery (Figure 9)
The common carotid artery runs
up along the anterior margin of
the sternocleidomastoid muscle. It
is enclosed by the cervical vertebral

Figure 8
The carotid artery

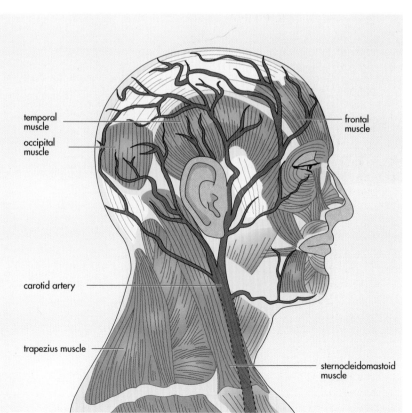

temporal muscle

occipital muscle

frontal muscle

carotid artery

trapezius muscle

sternocleidomastoid muscle

column and by the trachea and larynx. This artery supplies oxygen to the face, head, and back of the neck. If the muscles are contracted for a long time, the blood vessels become compressed; this restricts the oxygen supply, often resulting in tension headaches or facial pain.

At the level of the thyroid cartilage, the common carotid artery divides into the external and internal carotid arteries. The external carotid artery, or facial artery, primarily supplies the face, chewing muscles, tongue, pharynx, larynx, thyroid gland, and back of the neck with blood. The internal carotid artery runs inside the cranial cavity, where it supplies oxygenated blood to the eyes and, together with the vertebral artery, to the individual segments of the brain.

The vertebral artery runs upward from the sixth cervical vertebra through the foramina of the transverse processes and into the brain, where it supplies the cerebellum or posterior part of the brain with blood. When the muscles are constantly contracted or the head has poor posture, the carotid artery, which lies in the region of the powerful sternocleidomastoid muscle and other smaller muscles, is impaired.

In contrast, the vertebral artery depends primarily on the position of the cervical vertebrae. If the cervical vertebral column remains erect, the artery has enough room. If it is slanting, the blood vessels are compressed on one side. Bone attrition and degenerative changes, such as the formation of marginal serrations, can become problems.

The muscles of the neck

All the muscles attached to the head and neck joints can move the head and neck. However, the neck muscles also help in chewing and swallowing, as well as in moving the larynx.

Bending the head and cervical vertebral column forward

The deep or prevertebral musculature (lying directly in front of the spinal column) is responsible for bending the head (Figure 10):

- Long muscle of the neck: With bilateral contraction, it lifts the cervical concave curve and bends the cervical vertebral column.
- Long muscle of the head
- Rectus capitis anterior muscle

The upper cervical vertebral column is bent by the long head muscles and the rectus capitis anterior muscles in the upper head joint.

Figure 9
The vertebral artery and the carotid artery

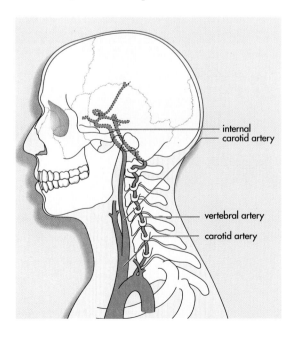

internal
carotid artery

vertebral artery

carotid artery

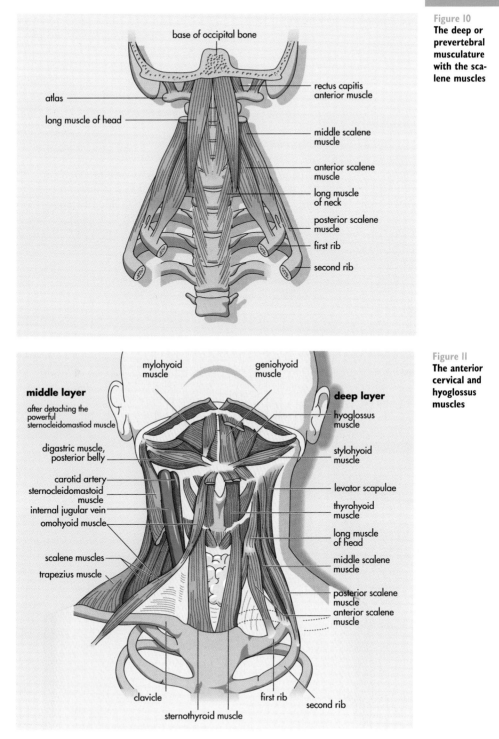

Figure 10
The deep or prevertebral musculature with the scalene muscles

base of occipital bone

atlas

long muscle of head

rectus capitis anterior muscle

middle scalene muscle

anterior scalene muscle

long muscle of neck

posterior scalene muscle

first rib

second rib

Figure 11
The anterior cervical and hyoglossus muscles

mylohyoid muscle

geniohyoid muscle

middle layer

after detaching the powerful sternocleidomastiod muscle

deep layer

hyoglossus muscle

digastric muscle, posterior belly

carotid artery
sternocleidomastoid muscle
internal jugular vein
omohyoid muscle

stylohyoid muscle

levator scapulae

thyrohyoid muscle

long muscle of head

scalene muscles

trapezius muscle

middle scalene muscle

posterior scalene muscle
anterior scalene muscle

clavicle

first rib

second rib

sternothyroid muscle

The long neck and head muscles provide for movement in the successive joints.

The long muscle of the head, located directly in front of the spinal column, is very important for the equilibrium of the cervical vertebral column. With simultaneous contraction of the anterior cervical and posterior splenius muscles, it becomes fixed in its midposition. With unilateral contraction of a cervical muscle, the neck leans toward that side.

The scalene muscles also bend the head to the side if they are contracted unilaterally. Since they originate from the transverse processes of the cervical vertebrae and extend to the first two ribs, if the cervical vertebral column is held in place, they can raise the two upper ribs, acting as part of the breathing mechanism. Although the scalene muscles participate in bending the cervical vertebral column, they reinforce the cervical concavity, if the column is not maintained by the long muscle of the neck.

In contrast, the inferior hyoglossal muscles help bend the head and cervical vertebral column while they simultaneously reduce the cervical concavity. For this reason, they are also important for the equilibrium of the cervical vertebral column (Figure 11).

> **The musculature of the anterior cervical and posterior splenius muscles acts as a brace. Obviously, the equilibrium between the two is lost if one muscle side is too weak or shortened.**

Bending the head and cervical vertebral column backward

Bending the head backward involves the musculature of the back of the neck, consisting of four superpositioned layers.

The short muscles of the back of the neck

This deep muscle layer lies directly on the skeleton. It connects the occiput (the back of the head), the atlas, and the axis. The short muscles that act on the head joints make precise graduated movements of the head possible; however, for most people these muscles are tense or shortened because of poor head posture.

They can flex the head back or, if contracted unilaterally, bend or turn the head to the side.

The short muscles of the back of the neck are the following:
- Rectus capitis posterior minor muscle

Figure 12
The deep muscles of the back of the neck

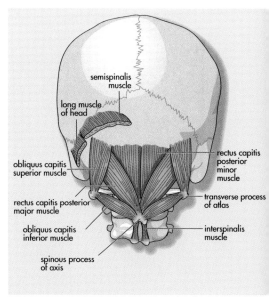

semispinalis muscle

long muscle of head

obliquus capitis superior muscle

rectus capitis posterior major muscle

obliquus capitis inferior muscle

spinous process of axis

rectus capitis posterior minor muscle

transverse process of atlas

interspinalis muscle

- Rectus capitis posterior major muscle
- Superior oblique muscle of the head
- Inferior oblique muscle of the head

The cervical portion of the spinal erector

The transversospinal system functions as part of the spinal erector, forming a long muscular tract to the right and left of the spinal column. It originates at the axis; its continuing muscle bundles extend to the sacrum. The numerous large and small muscles that make up the spinal erector support the spinal column as a whole. Individually, they are attached to the spinous and transverse processes and fill in the space between them (Figure 13).

The cervical portion of this muscle system can cause the cervical vertebral column to be too concave, straighten it, or, when contracted on one side, rotate it.

The deep tract of this middle muscle bundle of the spinal erector includes:
- Rotator muscles
- Multifidus muscles
- Semispinalis muscle (in pairs)
- Dorsal sternocleidomastoids

While the muscles in the deep layers run only from segment to segment, the muscles in the superficial layers are longer. The most powerful muscle groups are located in the region of the cervical and lumbar concavity.

The superficial bundle of this muscle layer consists of only long muscle tracts:
- Long muscles of the neck and head
- Iliocostalis muscle (cervical portion)
- Splenius cervicis and splenius capitis muscles

While the muscles have an important posture function for the spinal column and are in part responsible for holding it erect, they can also

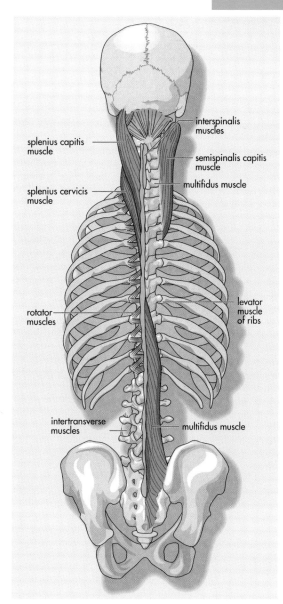

splenius capitis muscle

splenius cervicis muscle

rotator muscles

intertransverse muscles

interspinalis muscles

semispinalis capitis muscle

multifidus muscle

levator muscle of ribs

multifidus muscle

Figure 13
The spinal erector muscles

Figure 14
The muscles of the shoulder girdle

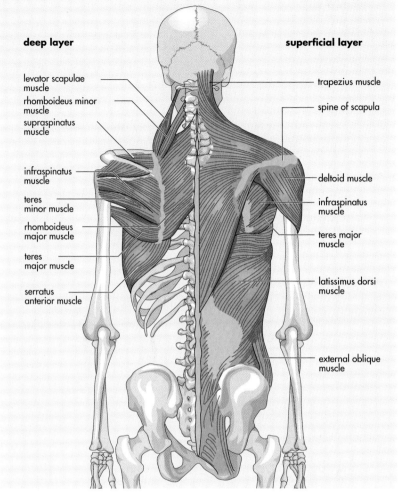

deep layer

levator scapulae muscle

rhomboideus minor muscle

supraspinatus muscle

infraspinatus muscle

teres minor muscle

rhomboideus major muscle

teres major muscle

serratus anterior muscle

superficial layer

trapezius muscle

spine of scapula

deltoid muscle

infraspinatus muscle

teres major muscle

latissimus dorsi muscle

external oblique muscle

flex the cervical vertebral column backward; if contracted unilaterally, the splenius muscles help rotate the head.

Superficial layer of the muscles of the back of the neck

The superficial layer primarily controls the upper extremities. It is responsible for moving the arms and shoulders (Figure 14). The layer consists of:

• Levator scapulae: This is located close to the splenius muscle and is for the most part covered by the trapezius. Its most powerful point of attachment is the atlas. Its sinewy fibers end at the superior angle of the scapula. The levator scapulae supports the trapezius. If the cervical vertebral column is held in place, the levator scapulae raises the shoulder blade forward and upward. On the other hand, if the shoulder blade is stationary, the muscle exerts a stretching and concave action on the cervical vertebral column.

- Trapezius: The superficial layer of the neck muscles is formed by the trapezius (Figure 15). Parts of this muscle make a profound impression on the contour of the lower side of the neck. It connects the occiput (the back of the head) with the shoulder girdle and acts on the shoulder girdle and shoulder blade.

  If the shoulder girdle is held in place, the trapezius pulls back the cervical vertebral column and head to produce concavity. If the anterior cervical muscles are contracted at the same time, the trapezius, just like the levator scapulae, functions as a tensioning rope that stabilizes the cervical vertebral column. If we compare the spinal column to the mast of a ship, the back muscles, including the muscles of the back of the neck, represent the tension cables that hold the mast perpendicular.

- Sternocleidomastoid muscle: It actually belongs to the superficial musculature of the ventral side of the neck. Only the cervical cutaneous muscle overlaps it. However, it works together with the muscles of the back of the neck.

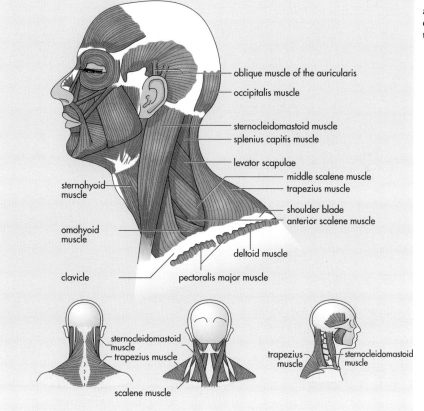

Figure 15
The trapezius and stern-ocleidomas-toid muscles

oblique muscle of the auricularis

occipitalis muscle

sternocleidomastoid muscle
splenius capitis muscle

levator scapulae

middle scalene muscle
trapezius muscle

shoulder blade
anterior scalene muscle

sternohyoid muscle

omohyoid muscle

deltoid muscle

clavicle

pectoralis major muscle

sternocleidomastoid muscle
trapezius muscle

trapezius muscle

sternocleidomastoid muscle

scalene muscle

These muscles and the two sternocleidomastoid muscles ensure that the head remains perfectly balanced on the spinal column and is in equilibrium. Each sternocleidomastoid muscle connects the cranium with the anterior part of the shoulder girdle and sternum. It traverses the cervical vertebral column, originates at two heads—one sternal and one clavicular—and runs upward at an oblique angle to the neck until it attaches to the mastoid process of the temporal bone. Contracting one of the sternocleidomastoid muscles bends the cervical vertebral column to that side or rotates the head to the opposite side. Simultaneous contraction of the two muscles lifts the head or tilts it back. If the cervical concavity is offset or prevented by other muscles, both sternocleidomastoid muscles can flex the cervical vertebral column.

Muscular equilibrium in the neck region

The purpose of the retaining muscles is to keep the skeleton erect. In the neck region, many different muscles stabilize the neck so that the head can rest in equilibrium erect or even relaxed.

The considerable difference in strength between the ventral flexor muscles and the dorsal extensor muscles makes it easy to pull the head back. In addition, the dorsal muscles prevent the head from falling forward.

The small cervical muscles are especially susceptible to strains

when they are overtaxed by poor head posture. You can usually feel this painful strain where the muscles attach to the cranium. The points where muscles attach are by far the most susceptible to painful and chronic strains.

The longer you stay in an asymmetric posture (for example, at a desk or computer or at a machine), the longer certain muscles will remain contracted. When you lean over or bend your head down, the muscles in the back of the neck are involved. Gradually, they become harder until they form knots, or myogeloses.

Muscle strains are also frequent causes of back pain that can be very persistent. The muscles of the back of the neck can be compared to the supporting wires of a flag pole-if one is stiff or shortened, the pole bends.

When the muscles of the back of the neck are too stiff and impair healthy joint mobility, they pull the cervical vertebrae forward; when a lateral cervical muscle bundle is too

There is only one way to overcome muscle strains:

- Become aware of your body—to learn to distinguish poor head posture from good posture and to prevent continuous contractions

- Stretch—to loosen cramps and get the blood in the contracted tissue flowing again

- Strengthen—to prepare and strengthen weak muscles to stabilize the cervical vertebral column

tight, it bends the cervical vertebral to one side. The muscular equilibrium is then completely disturbed, and the head isn't balanced, so it cannot hang freely.

Primarily, it is the large muscles of the neck that initiate movements of the head. However, this means that the smaller muscles of the back of the neck, which attach to the occipital joint, become atrophied, shortened, and strained.

In addition, straining a muscle disturbs the flow of blood to the area. The muscles don't receive enough fresh, oxygen-rich blood; and the blood trapped in the contracted tissue has too much carbon dioxide. The metabolic waste products are not all carried off, and they accumulate in the muscles.

A vicious cycle begins: Pain in the back of the neck causes you to hold your head even more rigidly, and this posture only increases the tension.

Muscular equilibrium in the shoulder girdle

Shifts in balance generally affect the neck region. Since most people work with their arms in a forward position, they use their chest and neck muscles extensively.

This posture pulls up the shoulders, increasing strains. It may also shorten the levator scapulae muscles. At the same time, the muscles that pull the shoulder blades down become weaker.

Instead of moving our arms only from the shoulder joints, we have shifted the movement process to the shoulder blade, although this is not necessary.

Thus, we use the muscles of the back of the neck (the upper trapezius muscles) for every hand and arm movement. These muscles rarely get any rest, while the actual arm abductors (deltoid and supraspinatus muscles) atrophy.

For this reason, we should pay attention to when and how often we pull our shoulders up, such as when we put the telephone receiver to our ear, drink a cup of coffee, or get something from a high shelf or cabinet. Even when we lift our arms, we should not lift our shoulders with them.

A general rule of posture that produces muscular balance in the shoulder, neck, and back of the neck:

- **Chin back**
- **Back of the neck long**
- **Shoulders low**

Posture and its significance

Our posture is influenced by several factors:

- Skeletal equilibrium (shape of the spinal column)
- Psyche (feeling anxious, upset, overwhelmed, cheerful, or strong)
- Muscle functions (muscular balance or imbalance)
- Mobility of joints
- Flexibility or stability of ligaments

Biomechanically proper posture

For human beings, there is a biomechanically proper posture and an improper posture; we could also call these a back-friendly posture and an unfriendly posture. Posture is just as much an expression of our personality and emotional state at any given moment as it is the result of stress on our locomotor system.

We can perform each movement economically, meaning with the smallest possible expenditure of effort for the greatest possible effect. The farther our posture moves from the biomechanically proper, the less possible it is for movement to be economical. The ideal posture places minimum stress on the knees, muscles, ligaments, and intervertebral disks.

We are constantly exposed to earth's gravity and must maintain an erect posture against it. Such an effort requires a substantial muscular output. The question is, how we can maintain an erect posture most economically, that is, with the smallest possible expenditure of effort, against gravity.

If we compare the body to a building, it can be either stable or unstable. Stability is ensured if a body is perpendicular to the ground. The plumb line always goes through the body's center of gravity (Figure 16). The farther a body part is from the plumb line, the more muscle force is necessary to maintain the perpendicular so that we do not fall over.

However, we do not exist in a stable equilibrium, but in an unstable one, because the body's center of gravity shifts whenever we move or change position. If we bend forward just a little, the body's center of gravity shifts forward.

The earth's gravity and torque affect us. To prevent the body from falling over, the dorsal muscles contract. When we bend forward, they contract even more.

If the head is bent forward for too long or the cervical vertebral column is pushed too far forward, that is, if it is in front of the plumb line for a long time, the muscles of the back of the neck must do considerably more work to prevent the head from yielding to the downward pull of gravity. The dorsal muscles are thus continuously contracted.

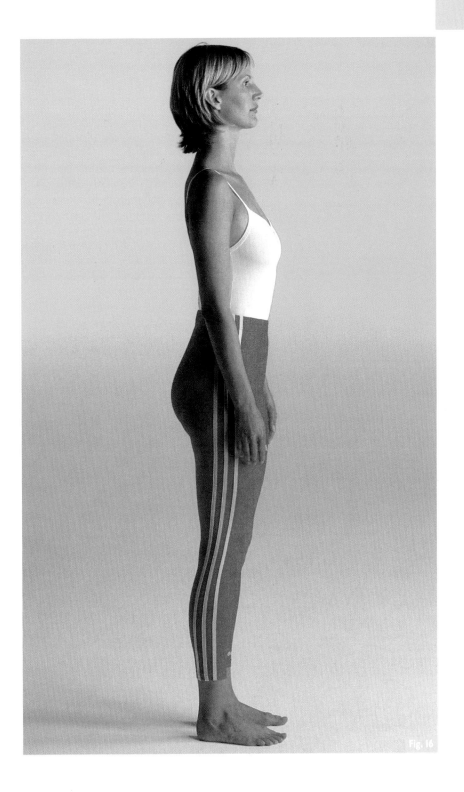

Fig. 16

If the body is balanced, the center of gravity is located somewhere between the navel and the fourth lumbar vertebra. In the erect state, the plumb line runs from the outer ear canal through the shoulder, hip, and knee joints to the floor just in front of the ankle. It passes the seventh cervical, twelfth thoracic, and fifth lumbar vertebrae.

If one body part falls outside the perpendicular, the neighboring spinal column segments must change their positions in order to restore an artificial balance. Thus, pushing the cervical vertebral column forward usually results in a humpback in the thoracic vertebral column area and a hollow back farther down (Figure 17).

In our culture, we typically find that a pulled-back head accompanies a pushed-forward cervical vertebral column. This is especially true for those who sit a lot at a desk or computer, but also at a drawing board, in a factory, or at a cash register. When we sit at a table or desk, we almost always lean our heads back if we are viewing a distant object or want to talk with someone next to or somewhat removed from us (Figure 18). This places particular stress on the uppermost head joint (occipital joint) between the cranium and the atlas because it is forced to cope with an extreme position for a long time. However, this position also subjects the transition between cervical and thoracic vertebral columns (seventh cervical vertebra) to intense stress and strain. Years of assuming such a head posture frequently results in a small "hump" in this region. Moreover, constrictions develop between the cervical vertebrae, compressing the nerve exit points and blood vessels in this segment.

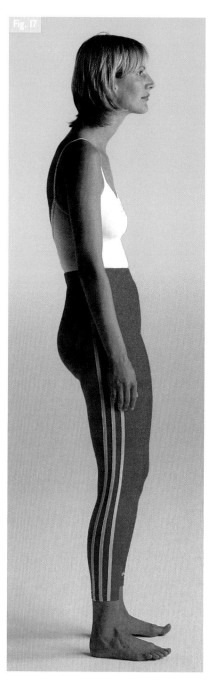

Fig. 17

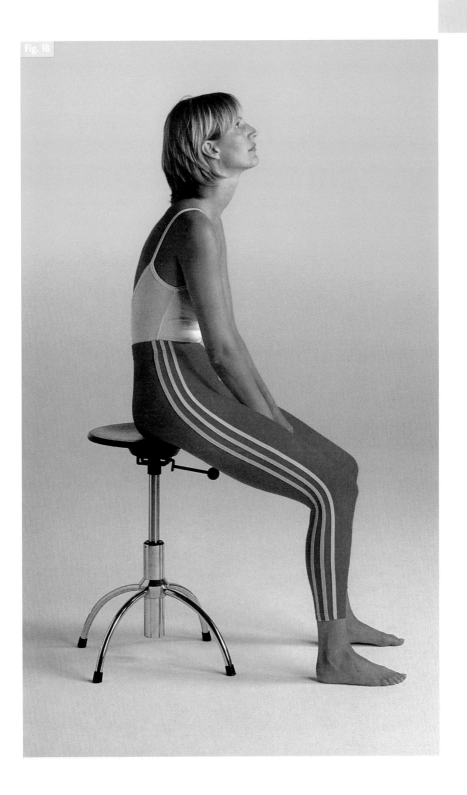

Fig. 18

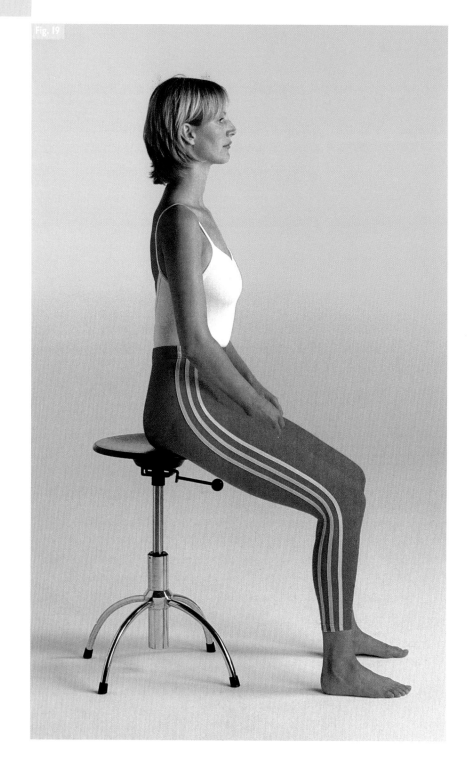

Fig. 19

Over the years, constant improper posture of the cervical vertebral column and head gradually becomes the normal condition for the head joint. The brain also gradually interprets this posture as "normal." The result is degenerative and sometimes inflammatory changes in the connective tissue inside individual segments and in the accompanying muscle fasciae (the sheets of tissue that surround muscle). This is true for both the small vertebral arch joints and the intervertebral disks.

Therefore, we must first become aware of our own posture and understand the dangers of over-stressing individual body parts (muscles, ligaments, joints, disks) and the dangers of understressing others (weakening).

Balancing the head

The head is heavy—after all, it weighs 15 to 16 pounds (7kg). Its center of gravity is located in front of the cervical vertebral column. Because the anterior part (visceral cranium) is heavier than the posterior part, the cervical vertebral column is at risk of sagging forward. However, the powerful muscles of the back of the neck protect the head from toppling forward.

Indeed, in a posture in which the head is usually bent forward, the muscles of the back of the neck are typically thoroughly strained and forced to support the posture continuously. They become short and are no longer capable of relaxing.

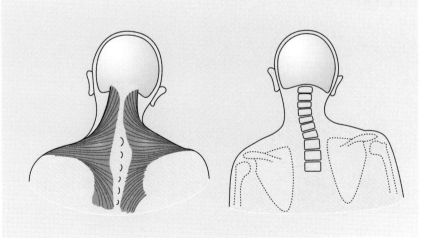

Figure 20
An imbalance of the cervical vertebral column causes asymmetric shortening and straining of the shoulder and neck muscles.

At the same time, the muscles that bend the neck and prevent the head from falling backward gradually atrophy. The head can only be evenly balanced in a relaxed manner on the cervical vertebral column when the anterior and posterior muscles are in equilibrium and work together.

On the other hand, imbalances lead to strains, faster wear, disturbances, and disorders. They frequently result from repetitive motion or habitual posture at work stations that permit little range of motion.

The cervical vertebral column can also bend to one side. One ear is then closer to the shoulder on that side than the other ear is to the other shoulder. Since one shoulder is somewhat higher than the other, the shoulder and neck muscles on one side are shorter and usually more cramped than on the other side (Figure 20). Asymmetrical movement, work patterns, and postures also cause this asymmetrical posture.

Susceptibility of the cervical vertebral column to injury and the consequences

The vertebrae tend to accumulate calcium on their boundary surfaces as they age. This can have negative consequences on the blood vessels and exiting nerves since more pressure is exerted on these vessels and nerves. Intervertebral disk injuries

and bone and joint attrition also generally increase with age. The vessels in the area of the neck become more constricted, choking off the blood supply to the brain and inner ear.

If we compound this condition by frequently assuming incorrect posture or extreme positions (for example, holding the telephone receiver between the ear and shoulder or working above head level hanging curtains or painting a ceiling), increasing muscular tension, we can develop headaches, migraines, dizziness, and a reduced supply of blood to the inner ear.

However, chronically increased muscular tension is also frequently caused by emotional problems. Stress, the pressure to achieve, the fear of failure or other anxieties, blind rage, or anger over an injustice often place a heavy burden on our shoulders.

Since the blood vessels and nerves within the muscle layers and in the intervertebral foramina are then constantly under pressure, we experience pain.

Chronic strain burdens us for the rest of our lives if we do not do something about it.

However, you can change:

With posture awareness, stretching, relaxing and breathing exercises, you can break out of the vicious cycle of tension, pain, and renewed tension. If you follow the program in this book, you can become healthy and stay healthy.

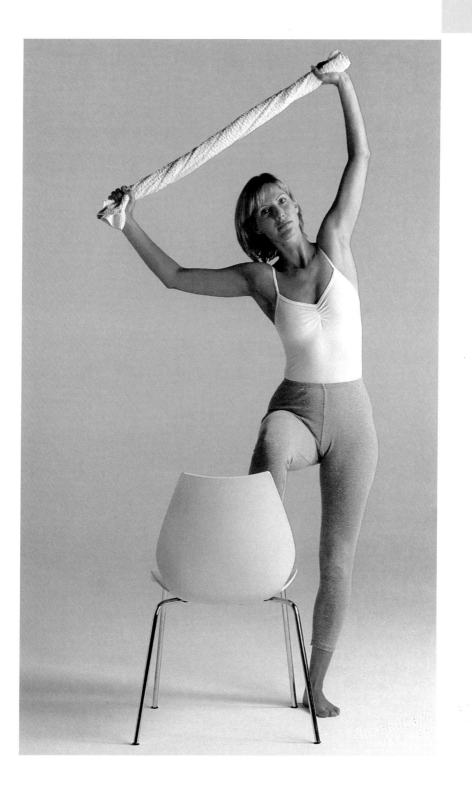

Neck training—the right way to do it

Warm-up exercises

Begin each exercise program with special exercises to warm up the entire body and prepare for the activity. Warm-up exercises ensure that the muscles, joints, tendons, and ligaments you want to train are well-supplied with blood and adequately prepared. A warmed-up muscle can be stretched and trained; a loosened joint can handle more stress than a "cold" one. This prevents injuries, such as pulls, and reduces muscle soreness. Moreover, exercises stimulate the heart and circulation. Suitable warm-up exercises include swinging and circling motions with the arms and shoulders, including pendulum swings, figure-eight swings, etc. Shaking movements with the arms or shoulders are also pleasant.

Body awareness and body sense

Most coordinated movements that we perform every day take place subconsciously and automatically. People develop their own unique coordinated movements. Whether we are walking, standing, sitting, moving, playing, eating, writing, doing housework, driving an automobile, or working on the computer, we always assume the same posture to perform our standardized coordinated movements.

For this reason, we must begin by retraining and redeveloping our own body sense. Then, we can also have better control throughout our daily routine and correct our posture.

Body consciousness assumes that we are capable of perceiving tension within our own body. Most people have lost this consciousness.

We no longer recognize uneconomical, harmful movements and postures. We retain our improper head posture or kyphotic (convex) posture in all situations; our strained shoulders must cope with continuous contraction.

For whatever reason, we have learned an incorrect posture, and we no longer perceive it as harmful. Instead, we believe it is normal. However, "normal" would be that after a muscle has carried out its proper contraction or stretching, it returns immediately to its starting position (base tension). This is no longer happening with continuous contraction.

> Recognize your individual posture and movement habits. Learn to turn harmful posture patterns into healthy ones. You need to rethink your posture. Think about it over and over, applying your new knowledge daily until the new posture and movement patterns become established and automatic.

The only way to change is to become sensitive to your body and its conditions. You must learn to listen to, feel, and touch your body deep down inside in order to recognize, distinguish, and correctly interpret both positive and negative movement patterns. After you recognize and become conscious of posture (body awareness), the next step is correcting your problems with exercises. The final step is to make the new posture "normal" or automatic by frequently repeating the posture and movement exercises.

> **Get to know your habitual head posture at work and in leisure activities. Correct it consciously in your everyday routine until the proper posture feels "normal."**

You'll find training exercises that establish an equilibrium of the neck and shoulder muscles in the "Exercise" chapter of this book.

Awareness exercises for the cervical vertebral column

These exercises will help you become aware of your posture. They'll also help you distinguish between your usual posture and the proper posture of the head and cervical vertebral column.

Basic exercise:
Sit on a chair, possibly in front of a table. Sit naturally, without exerting yourself or trying to sit properly. Allow your body to collapse a little, just as you do every day from

habit. Feel how your back becomes rounded and your cervical vertebral column moves forward.

Look up as if you wanted to observe something located next to or somewhat removed from you. Do you feel how this pulls the back of your head back and down (Figure 21)?

Consciously direct your attention to the base of your skull where the spinal column ends and rotates. The back of your head is pulled far back by the shortened small muscles of the back of the neck, as if you wanted to pull the

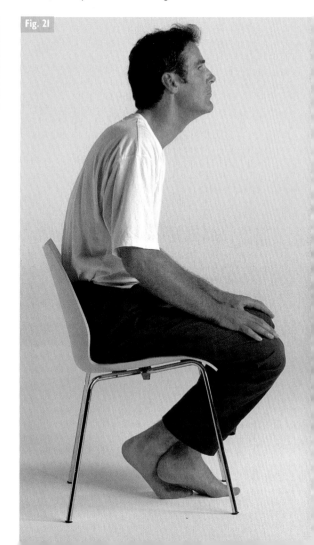

Fig. 21

back of your head between your shoulder blades.

Can you imagine how the small head and vertebral joints become worn down on one side? Notice how the front of the neck is over-stretched, while the back of the neck collapses and retracts.

Tip: Start by watching yourself in front of a mirror.

Sit up straight on the chair and imagine that you have a thread attached to the middle of the top of your head. Imagine that this thread is pulling you up to the ceiling, or imagine that you want to push a book that is on your head up to the ceiling (Figure 22). Do you feel how the back of your neck and your spinal column become extended? Let your shoulders hang down and feel how the

Fig. 22

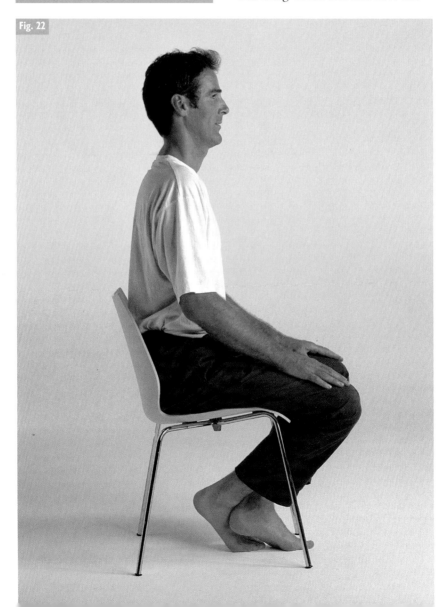

head posture and the head joints become freer.

However, be careful not to lift your chin or push your forehead toward the ceiling. Don't hold your chin too high or too low. Hold it so that you are looking straight ahead.

Additional awareness exercises:

- Feel your cervical vertebral column by placing your right middle finger in the recess in the lower middle of the back of your head. Slide the index finger of your left hand from this point over the vertebrae of the cervical vertebral column until it reaches the protruding seventh cervical vertebra (Figure 23). Repeat this touching-sliding movement a few times to become aware of your cervical vertebral column as an entity and also of its individual vertebrae.
- Place your right middle finger again in the recess in the middle of the back of your head. Place the fingers of your left hand on the spinous processes of the cervical vertebrae. Press the cervical vertebral column back against the fingers of this hand, hold that position for a few seconds before you press the cervical vertebrae forward (Figure 24). Become aware of the movement of the cervical vertebral column and feel how it extends and bends.
- Using the same finger position as above, incline your head to the right side, then to the left side (Figures 25 and 26). Become aware of the lateral movement of the cervical vertebral column.
- Allow yourself to sink down in the chair and lean your head

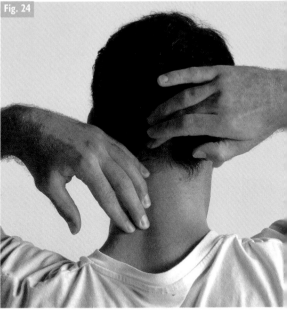

Fig. 23

Fig. 24

back. (You probably always sit like this without being aware of it). Place the fingers of one hand on the spinous processes of the cervical vertebrae. Push your

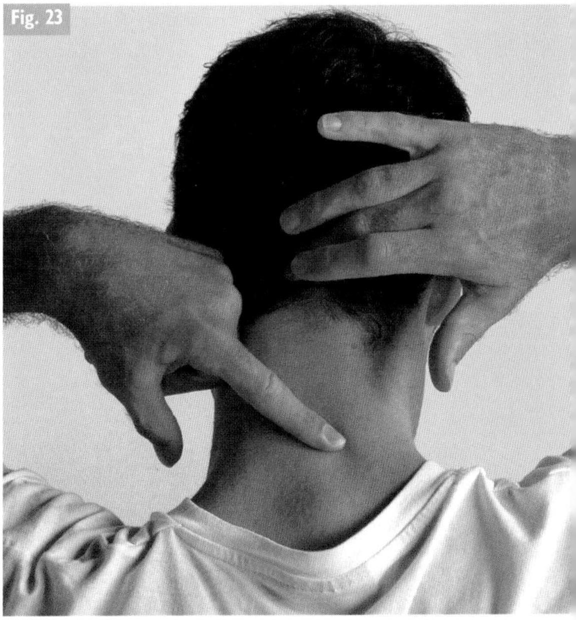

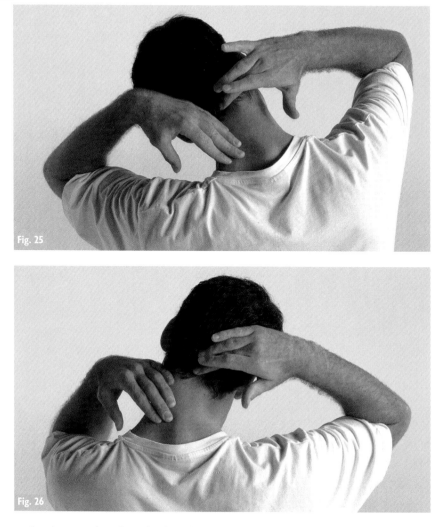

Fig. 25

Fig. 26

head upward as described in the basic exercise and feel the movement and change in the cervical vertebral column with your fingers.

Stretching and relaxing

Stretching basically means elongating a muscle through external forces so that the muscle becomes more flexible. Even with conscious (mental) relaxation alone, a shortened muscle can grow longer.

Of course, for a drastically shortened muscle, more intense stretching exercises are necessary. Bear in mind that a muscle will be elongated less by increasing the stretching tension than by yielding the muscle to the tension.

Muscles that have been shortened over a long period of time (for example, muscles that are continuously contracted), such as the muscles of the back of the neck, allow the connective tissue to form adhesions, and the tissue becomes inflexible. Stretching and relaxing makes the muscles supple and flexible. A shortened muscle no longer allows any free joint movement. However, before you embark on even a mild mobility program, you should first become aware of any tight muscles and then loosen them up. This sounds easier than it is because you may have lost the ability to "let go" or relax. Stress and the pressure to achieve eventually lead to internal and muscular tension. Even breathing is often constricted and superficial. Thus, you may have to relearn deep, relaxed breathing as well as relaxation. Tension reduces the elasticity of muscles, and shortened muscles subject the joint to which they are connected to substantially higher stress.

Relaxing and stretching increase both the elasticity and the metabolism of the muscle and the flexibility of the accompanying joint.

However, mobility also always means a loss of stability. For this reason, every exercise program should include strengthening exercises.

In addition to making you more mobile, stretching and relaxing make you "freer" and more relaxed, affecting even breathing and the head. Nerves and blood vessels are less compressed and jammed; they have more space and more oxygen.

Relaxing also means becoming aware of the weight of a body part or a body region. Experiencing the intrinsic weight allows you to develop body sense, and this is a prerequisite for relaxing. When you learn to feel the weight of your shoulder, you can let go of it and its increased contraction. It is helpful to experience and let go of the weight of each body part. This type of relaxing can elongate the muscles.

Breathing exercises also have a very relaxing effect. You can learn to exhale in every direction and to "send" the breath to all regions of the body, even to the most remote cell.

Conscious breathing supports stretching and makes the exercise easier and more effective. Observing your breathing has an additional relaxing effect.

Stretching methods

When stretching, you must take into account that the muscle reacts by contracting when you activate it or place it in a stretching position. The contraction is a reflex that protects the muscle from overstretching and tearing. With proper stretching, this initial contraction gives way to an easing of tension.

Passive static stretching

Slowly stretch the muscle up to the possible end point (the pain threshold) and hold the stretching position for 30 seconds or even longer. The initial stretching sensation always becomes weaker during the stretch because the contracting elements in the muscle fibers yield more and more to the tension. The stretching reflex, a jerky bouncing sensation that inhibits the stretch, begins immediately but ends after about 8 seconds. The tension slackens, and the muscles become more supple. This is usually perceived as a gentle "flowing apart" of the stretched muscle. At this point, you can easily intensify the stretching. Also at this point, you should not be experiencing any pain. Breathing can support the exercise.

- Example of an exercise for stretching the back of the neck: Tilt your head to the right side and notice the stretching tension on the left side of the neck. While slowly exhaling, let the weight of your head pull even more to the right and down. Trained individuals can concentrate on the left shoulder and let it drop lower while exhaling.
- The eyes can also intensify the effect in a reflexive way: Assume the position above, then while inhaling, look up and to the left with the eyes, while exhaling down and to the right. Let the weight of the head come into play.

Active static stretching

In active static stretching, you contract the antagonist of the muscles you want to stretch. This produces a reflexive inhibiting of the muscle so that the contracting muscle can perform more work, lowering the tension of the muscle so that you can stretch it more easily and effectively.

Postisometric relaxation

This type of stretching is also called simply contracting-relaxing stretching. It is the most effective type of stretching and produces a pronounced blood circulation and warming in the stretched muscle. It is generally acknowledged that a muscle which has experienced maximum contraction will then undergo maximum relaxation. At the end point of the stretch, the shortened (now stretched) muscle first experiences maximum isometric contraction (about 6 seconds) without any deflection of movement or shortening of the muscle. After a short relaxation interval (about 3 seconds) with the joint in the same position, gently stretch the muscle for a little longer. Hold the end position again for at least 10 seconds.

Strengthening

Muscles that are overstressed in relation to their capacity (frequently the back and neck muscles) are easily strained. Therefore, they must be strengthened. The same is true of muscles that are too weakly constructed in relation to their antagonists (frequently the abdominal muscles in contrast to the rather shortened and strained sacral muscles, or the cervical muscles in contrast to the neck muscles).

When a muscle is strengthened, it contracts. Shortening the muscles acts on the bones and can move them. Muscles act on joints as flexors and extensors. If one of these muscles on one side of a bone is shortened (for example, posterior neck muscles or sacral muscles), the opposite musculature (on the other side of the bone) is automatically lengthened.

You can stengthen muscles isotonically and isometrically. The isometric tension exercises, used intensely in the exercise programs for the neck and shoulder muscles, are more effective for training the retaining muscles. Scientists have shown that such exercises have the most intense effect within a short time. The ideal regimen combines isometric exercises and stretching exercises. You can find these in the "Exercise" chapter starting on page [40].

Isometric tension exercises

In isometric tension exercises, you slowly and forcefully contract a muscle against a resistance (for example, against your own hand or an object). This prevents muscle strains and activates as many muscle fibers as possible. Moreover, after a powerful muscle contraction, it is easier to control, perceive, and relax the muscle. Most experts agree that after a powerful muscle contraction, the relaxation can also be more intense.

Isometric muscle contraction means static retention work; the muscle develops tension without any change in length or articular movement. You can improve the stamina of your retaining muscles significantly. The isometric exercises have proven to be especially effective as an equalizing factor for the forced postures of the head which are often necessary in everyday life. They also work well for all neck and shoulder girdle problems as well as for fatigue, pain, and circulation disorders in the head region.

Be careful when exercising

- Always begin with warm-up exercises (perhaps to music).
- Be sure your starting position is back friendly (for example, sit or stand erect).
- Breathe evenly while exercising.
- Take your time with each exercise. If pressed for time, reduce the number of exercises. Perform each exercise slowly and deliberately.
- Never strain or pull a muscle!
- Never go beyond the pain threshold. If it hurts, stop.
- Perform the exercises with concentration and awareness. Listen to your body and feel what is happening inside it: during strengthening, stretching, and also during relaxing.
- Allow yourself time to feel the effect of an exercise: Has anything in the region of the body you were working on changed? How does this area feel now? How did it feel before the exercise?
- Remember, support the contraction by exhaling deeply. The most intense stretching is possible while exhaling. The best relaxing occurs with calm breathing and especially when exhaling deeply.

Performing isometric tension exercises: Maintain the muscle contraction for 6 to 10 seconds. During this time, breathe normally and evenly. Beginners must continue to remind themselves not to hold their breath or to compress their breath with the muscle contraction. Everyone who exercises should pay strict attention to breathing calmly. You need to consciously feel the contraction. Then, release the tension and consciously experience the relaxing. Repeat the sequence.

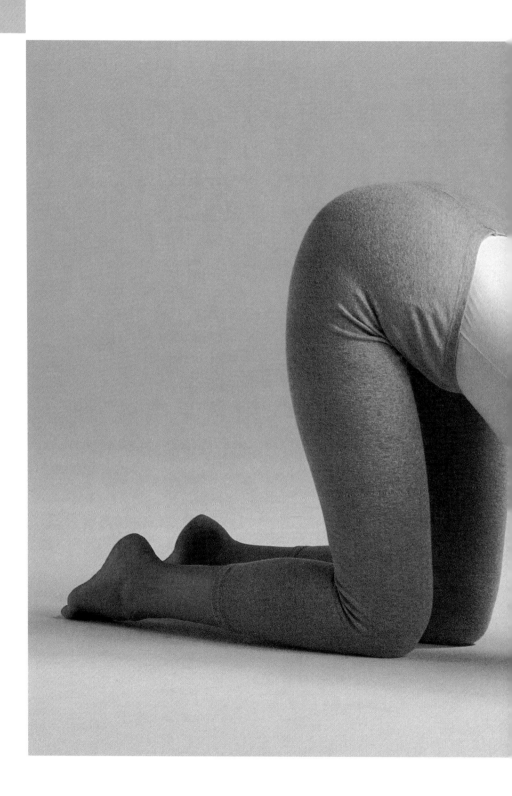

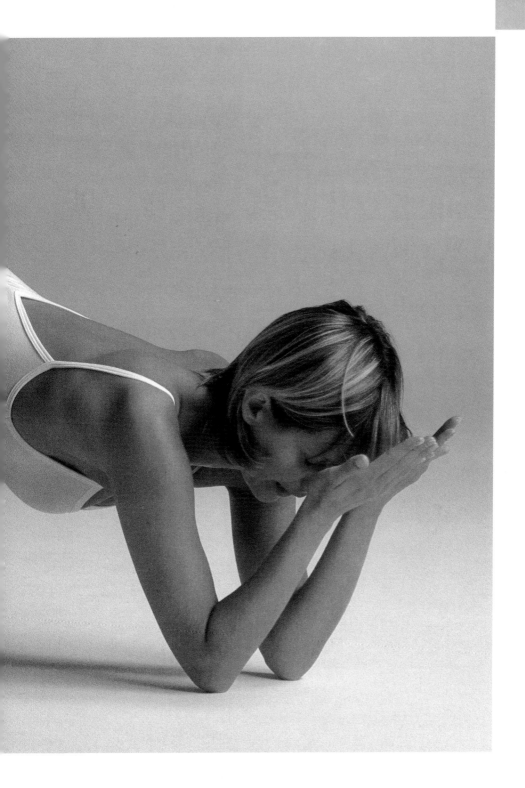

Exercise programs for the neck and shoulders

Exercise program I

Standing or sitting. A chair or large exercise ball is suitable for sitting.

Exercise I: Warm-up and awareness
• Warm-up: Shake your shoulders loosely and quickly by pulling them up fast and letting them drop again. This not only loosens you up, it also stimulates the circulation.

Swing your arms around like a jumping jack. Sit down and relax after you warm up. Feel the effect of the exercise.

Haven't your shoulder muscles become wonderfully warm?

> **This exercise is especially effective while bouncing on a large exercise ball.**

• Awareness: Consciously pull your shoulders up toward yours ears without using your arm muscles (Figure 27). Feel the contraction in the muscles. Allow your shoulders to drop heavily. Feel the relaxation in your shoulder and neck region (Figure 28). Keep your breathing calm and even.

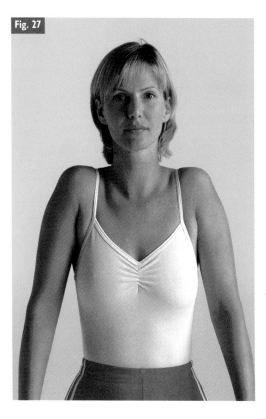

Fig. 27

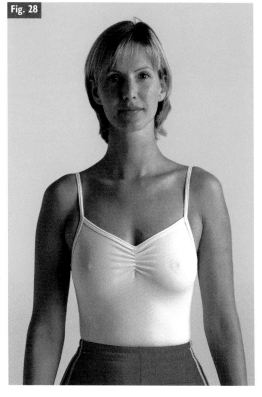

Fig. 28

Exercise 2: Massage

- Place the fingers of both hands on your hairline next to the spinal column. With some pressure, slide your hands along the spinal column from the top to the bottom until you reach your shoulders, continuing outward toward the shoulder joint (Figure 29). Repeat for as long as you want.
- As above, but use circular movements from top to bottom. Repeat this often.

Exercise 3: Posture

- Sit on a chair or large exercise ball. Imagine you are a marionette and you have a thread projecting from the middle of your skullcap. Act as if this thread could pull you up. The first few times, hold a few hairs between your fingers and gently tug on them (Figure 30). Notice how the cervical vertebral column and your entire back extend. Hold the position for 6 to10 seconds; relax, but don't collapse.

  Don't raise your chin; keep your shoulders down. A mirror will help you correct your posture during this exercise.

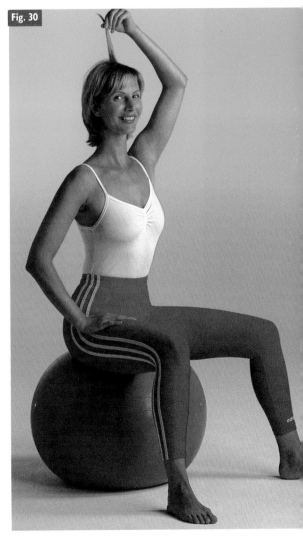

Fig. 30

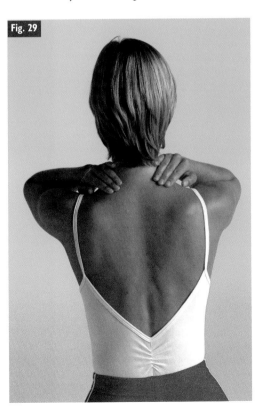

Fig. 29

Exercise 4: Strengthening

- Fold both hands and place them on the back of your head, or place one hand on the back of your head while the other supports the cervical vertebral column. Press the back of your head firmly against your hand for 6 to 10 seconds (Figure 31); relax. Perform the exercise four

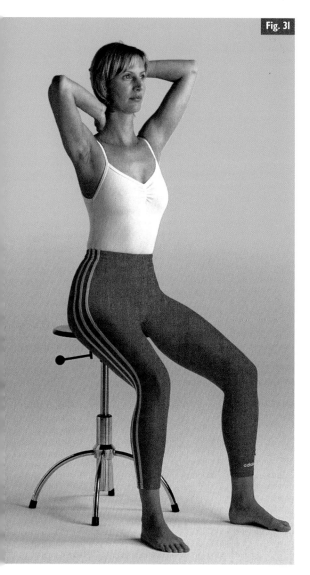

Fig. 31

to six times. Feel the stretch in your cervical vertebral column.

Exercise 5: Stretching and strengthening

- Place your hands as in Exercise 4, but bend your head forward (Figure 32). Feel the stretch, but don't press your head down. Press the back of your head against your hand for about 6 seconds without any motion.

    Relax and repeat the stretch. This time, use only the weight of your hand without pulling or straining. After a few repetitions, raise your head and concentrate on the relaxed and loose feeling you are experiencing.

Exercise 6: Mobility

- Place a finger in the recess at the back of the head. Try to push your finger back by pushing your chin back. Release the tension briefly before you contract again. Repeat, pushing the chin or finger back and releasing the tension a few times in succession.

    Try to feel your way into your upper head joint and upper vertebrae. Relax and concentrate on the loose feeling.

Exercise 7: Awareness, mobility, and loosening

- Place your middle fingers between both ears and the spinal column where the head joints are located. Make very small nodding movements up and down. Try again to feel your way into the saddle joint and imagine how the tip of your nose moves up and down with this small movement.

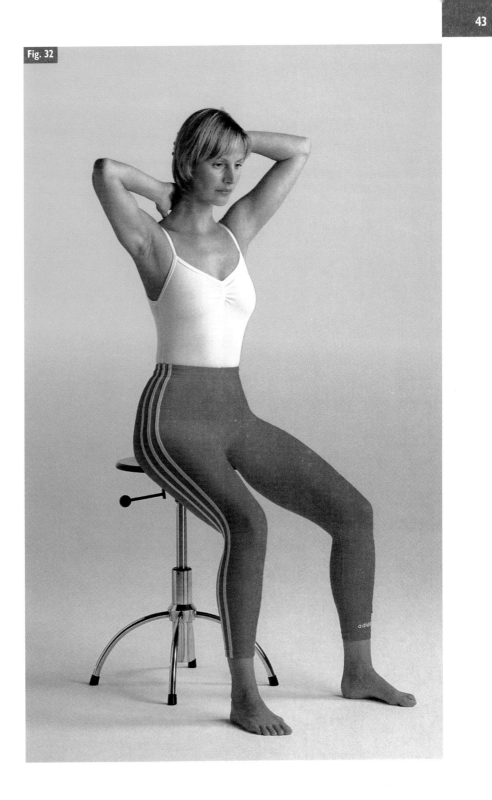

Fig. 32

Exercise program 2

Sitting on a stool in front of a wall. Push the stool against the wall.

Exercise I: Posture and stretching
- Sit on the stool in front of the wall so that your buttocks touch

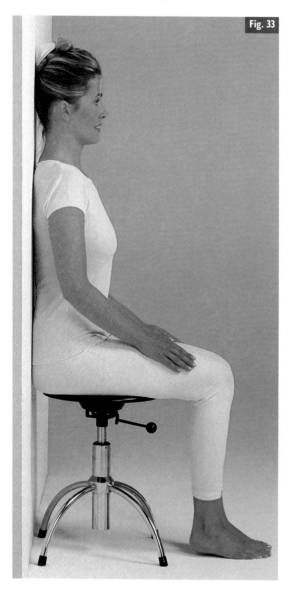

Fig. 33

the wall. Your hands should be resting on your thighs. Your shoulder region should be relaxed, but your shoulders should not slump forward. First, press your lower back firmly against the wall so that the convexity disappears and your back fits snugly to the wall (Figure 33). Do you feel how you have to tighten your abdominal muscles in this position?

Push the top of your head up

You might find it difficult to press the convexity against the wall. It is somewhat easier if someone else holds your heels to the floor in front of you at an oblique angle.

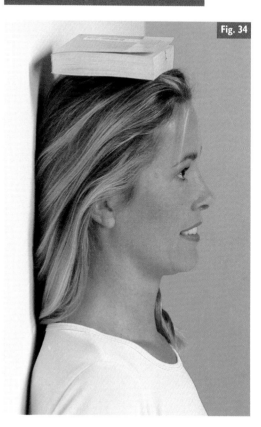

Fig. 34

and become aware of the stretching in the neck region. Do you feel how the stretching tension goes not only through the neck region, but also through the entire spinal column? Hold the stretch for 6 to 10 seconds; relax without collapsing. Repeat the exercise four to six times. If you need a little help, you can place a book on your head and push it toward the ceiling (Figure 34).

Exercise 2: Strengthening

- Use the same sitting posture as in Exercise 1. Once again, press your sacrum and shoulders against the wall. At the same time, push the back of your head up so that your neck extends. Notice the contraction in the anterior cervical region. Hold the tension for 6 to 10 seconds; relax. Repeat the exercise four to six times.

Exercise 3: Posture

- The same exercise as above, but let both arms hang down at your sides and against the wall. Press your sacrum and arms against the wall. Push the top of your head up while simultaneously pulling your arms and shoulders down (Figure 35). Hold the tension for 6 to 10 seconds while continuing to breathe normally.

Exercise 4: Stretching

- The same sitting position as above. As in Exercise 3, push the top of your head up and both arms and shoulders down (Figure 36). Tilt your head to the right side so that your right ear approaches your right shoulder (Figure 37). Look straight ahead or simply close your eyes to concentrate even better on

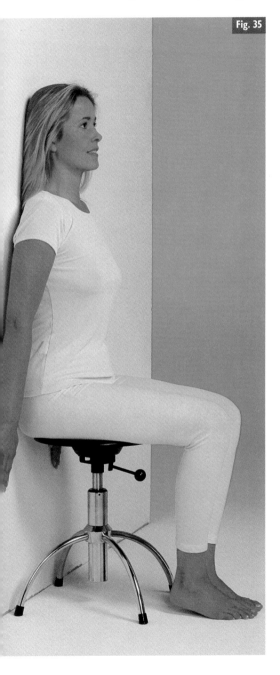

Fig. 35

what is happening in your body. Hold the stretching tension for 30 seconds while continuing to breathe normally; slowly return your head to its starting position until it once again rests erect on the spinal column. Concentrate on the feeling for a moment before you switch to the other side (Figure 38). Stretch each side two to three times.

This classic exercise for stretching the back of the neck, which has an especially positive effect on the levator scapulae muscles, can be performed anywhere, even while taking a break at your desk. It is useful for everyone because all of us generally contract or pull up our shoulders much too often. Exercising against a wall automatically leads to the correct upright posture.

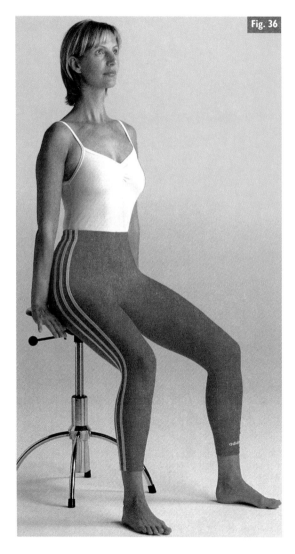

Fig. 36

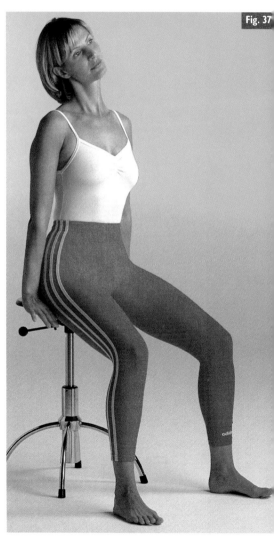

Fig. 37

During this stretching exer-cise, draw your chin gently toward your body in order to prevent hyperextension. Move your ear toward your shoulder so that your head moves down in a vertical line. Your head should not be rotated to the side.

- Perform the exercise as above but pull the opposite arm down, too (Figure 39). If your head is tilted to the right side, your left hand is pulled toward the floor. Consciously push the left shoul-der down with it; this intensifies the stretching in the shoulder region.

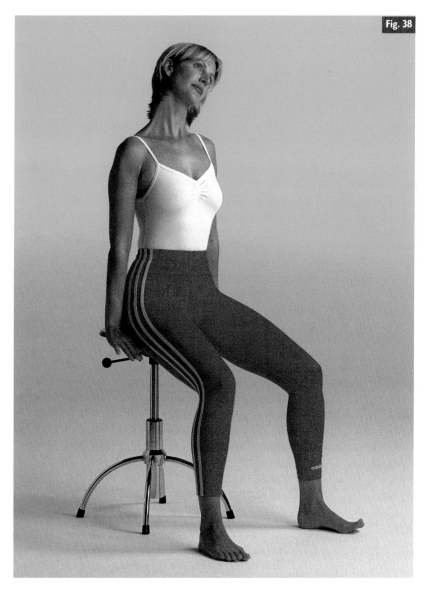

Fig. 38

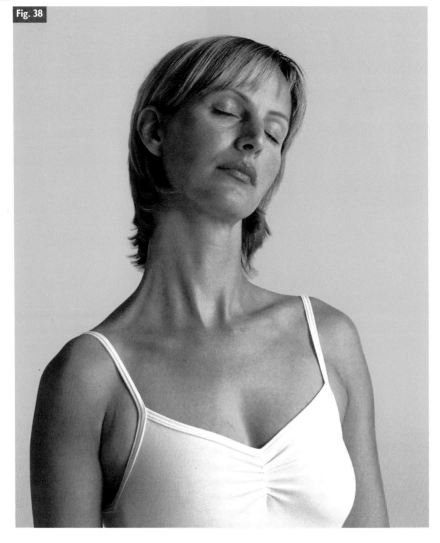

Fig. 38

Exercise 5: Mobility

- Sit with your back against a wall, raise both arms to your sides at shoulder height, and extend your arms. Press your sacrum against the wall. Then, press your arms against the wall and pull the top of your head up. Turn your head to the right so that the back of your head is about 1 inch (2cm) from it.

Turn your head as far as you comfortably can and look at your right hand. Hold the tension for 6 to 10 seconds before returning your head to the starting position in a relaxed manner. Lower your arms and relax briefly. Perform the same exercise on the other side. Repeat two to four times per side.

Exercise program 3

Standing or sitting.

Exercise I: Massage and warm-up

- Massage: Pass your hand over your neck to your shoulders, from top to bottom, as you learned in Exercise 2 of the first exercise program.
- Warm-up: Place your left hand over your right shoulder and feel for the muscle with your fingers (Figure 40). Pull it up and away from the shoulder between your fingers and the ball of your thumb. Hold it there for 4 to 6 seconds. Gently, let it slide back into place and concentrate on relaxing for a while. Repeat three to four times; switch sides.

(Tap the left muscle with the finger pads of the right hand and vice versa (Figure 41). Concentrate on the sensation. How does this area feel now?

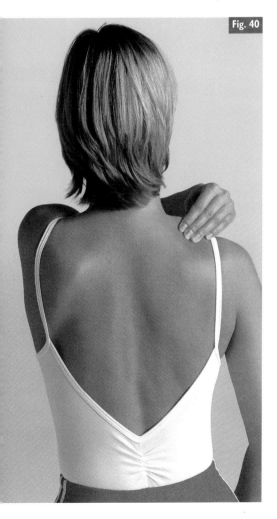

Fig. 40

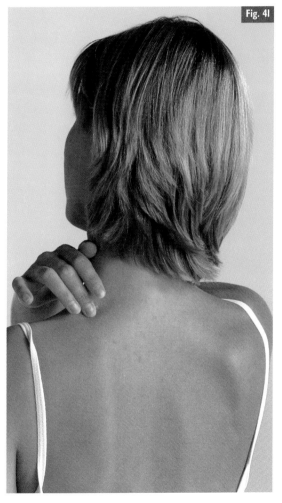

Fig. 41

Exercise 2: Awareness and relaxation

- Draw your right shoulder to your ear and feel the contraction in the shoulder region. At the same time, tilt your head to the right side so that the left side of your neck is stretched. The exercise becomes even more intense if you pull your left arm down toward the floor (Figure 42). After 6 to 10 seconds, let your shoulder and head return to the starting position and concentrate on the feeling.

The relaxation spreads to the shoulder girdle, the neck, and through the entire body. Switch sides (Figure 43); train each side two to four times. While exercising, continue to breathe normally, or exhale while drawing the shoulder up and inhale while releasing the tension.

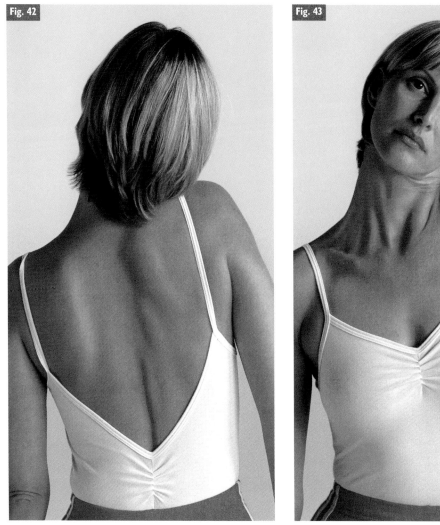

Fig. 42

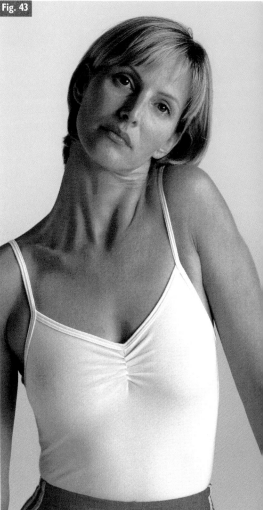

Fig. 43

Exercise 3: Strengthening

- Be sure to keep a straight, erect posture and let your arms hang down heavily. Turn your arms to the outside so that the palms of your hands face outward (Figure 44). Become aware of the movement of your shoulder blades.

  Draw them in even closer to the spinal column to strengthen the often weakened muscle. During this process, your head remains erect, and your arms always pull slightly to the outside in order to relieve the upper shoulder muscles. Do you feel the stretching in your chest muscles? After 6 to 10 seconds, return to the starting position, relax, and concentrate.

- As above, but continue to move your arms somewhat higher until they are almost in the horizontal position.

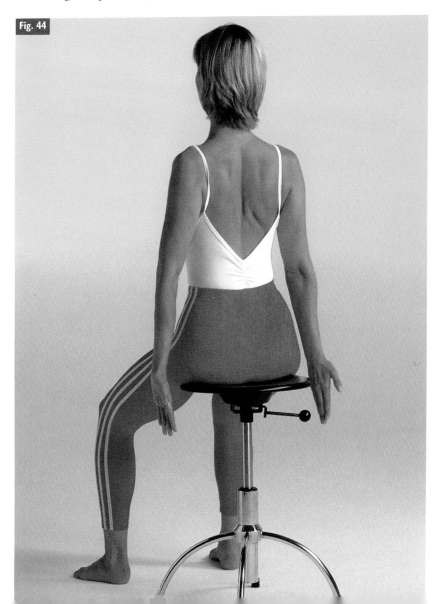

Fig. 44

Exercise 4: Strengthening and stretching

- Place the backs of both hands below your chin. This exercise is even better if you form a fist with the lower hand and put the other hand flat on top of it.

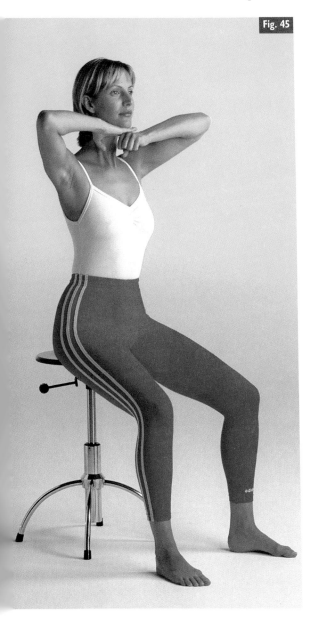

Fig. 45

Press your chin down forcefully against your hands (Figure 45). When performing this exercise concentrate on extending your neck.

Do not raise your shoulders. Hold the tension for 6 to 10 seconds before relaxing. Repeat four to six times.

- Stretching and strengthening: As above, press your chin against your hands. Alternate tilting your head to the right and left, moving your ear in the direction of your shoulder (Figure 46). Hold for 6 to 10 seconds for each side before returning your head to the erect position.

Exercise 5: Mobility and warm-up

- Start by placing your index finger in the recess of the back of your head where the spinal column joins your head. Concentrate on this point and make very small nodding movements up and down.

  Rotate your head slowly to the right and left so that you are first looking over the right shoulder, then over the left one.

  When you have become familiar with the nodding movement, you can remove your finger and put your hands down in a relaxed manner.

- Place one hand below your chin and make the nodding movement, as above, slowly to the right and left. Your hand now offers some resistance.

  Even if you have to concentrate, continue to breathe naturally. Pay attention to the sensation.

Fig. 46

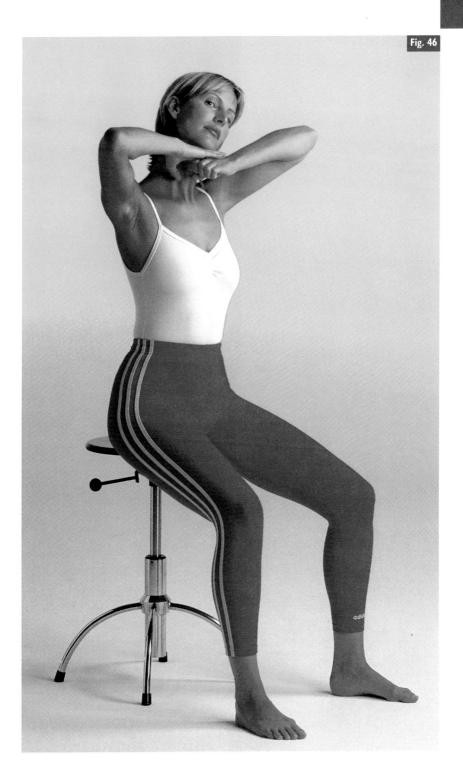

Exercise 6: Massage the small neck muscles

- Place your fingers on top of the back of your head with your thumbs on your hairline behind the ears. Make circular motions with your thumbs while gradually moving them along the hairline to the spinal column (Figures 47 and 48). Stop at as many points as possible along the way and make small circular motions. Feel free to exert pressure with your thumbs. This massages important acupressure points, loosening the small neck muscles. It also helps relieve headaches.

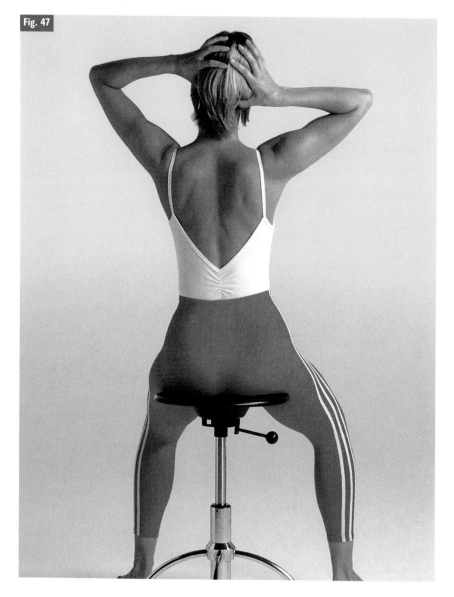

Fig. 47

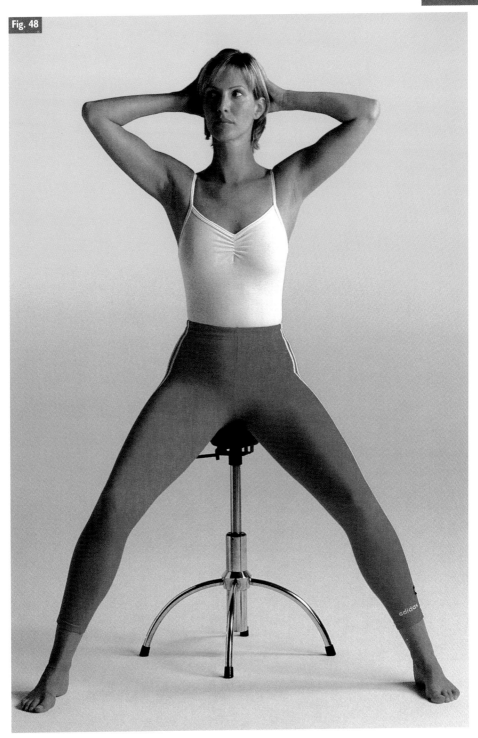

Fig. 48

Exercise program 4

Standing and sitting. You will need a towel rolled up lengthwise.

Exercise I: Breathing, posture, and awareness
- Breathing: Hold the rolled up towel high above your head with your hands at both ends. Pull slightly with both hands and inhale through your nose (Figure 49). Lower your arms, bringing the towel down in front of you, and slowly exhale through your mouth (Figure 50). Repeat four to six times.

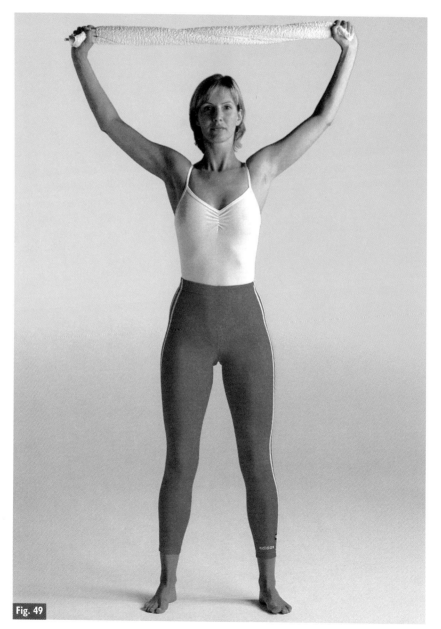

Fig. 49

- Posture and awareness: Raise the towel above your head and hold it there. This time consciously pull your shoulders down.

  Notice how the muscles between your shoulder blades contract while your neck muscles relax. Continue to breathe normally in this position for about 10 seconds. Push your arms up like antennae, inhale, pull your shoulders back down, and exhale slowly. Continue to breathe normally. Finally, lower your arms in a relaxed fashion. Perform the exercise a total of four to six times.

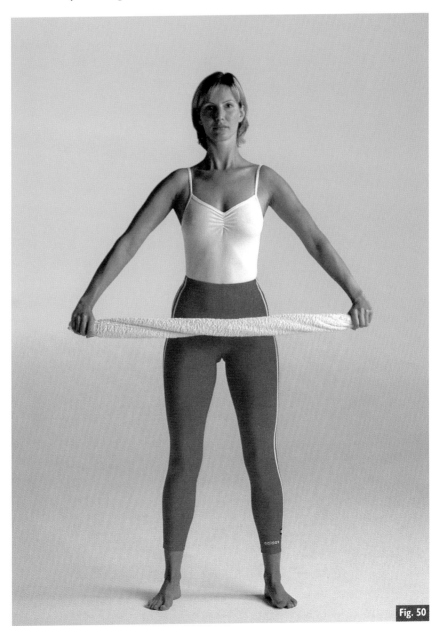

Fig. 50

Exercise 2: Massaging the small neck muscles

- Hold the rolled up towel at about shoulder height. Let the ends simply hang. Pull the towel back and forth behind your head in small, fast movements so that you massage and loosen up the occipital region, which is usually very tense (Figure 51). You can also move the towel up and down. Now and then, shake and loosen up your arms. You can perform this exercise for as long as you want, but afterward, allow yourself enough time to concentrate on the pleasant feeling in the upper neck region.

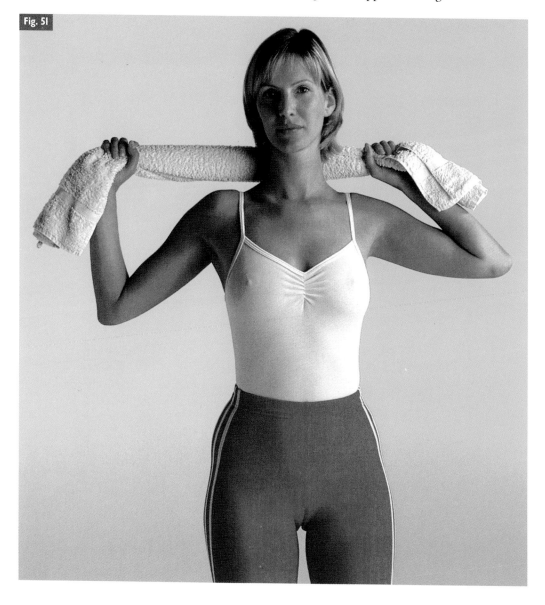

Fig. 51

Exercise 3: Increasing mobility and warming up the head joints

After you have massaged the area, suffusing the small neck muscles and the head joints with blood, the following exercise is helpful.

Imagine you have a pencil attached to the tip of your nose, or hold a pencil between your front teeth. Use it to draw figures in the air in front of you (Figure 52):

- Small circles, clockwise and counterclockwise
- Horizontal lines
- Vertical lines
- Zigzag lines
- Diagonal lines
- Horizontal figure eights
- Vertical figure eights
- Spirals (in the shape of a snail shell)
- Several interconnected roof tiles (turn your face both to the right and left)
- Your name
- Pictures or objects

This exercise works best if you close your eyes. Occasionally, direct your concentration to the uppermost vertebrae or to the head joints.

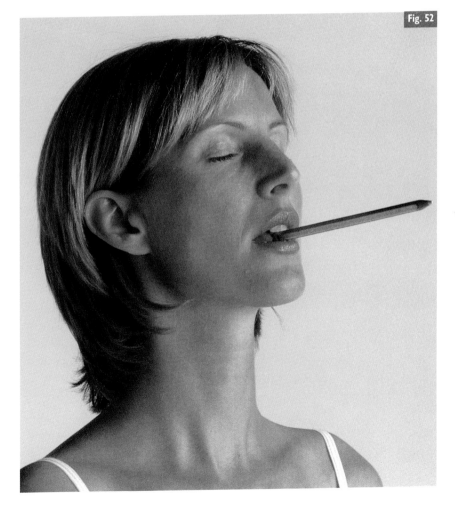

Fig. 52

Exercise 4: Strengthening

- Fold both hands and place them on the back of your neck. Forcefully press the cervical ver-

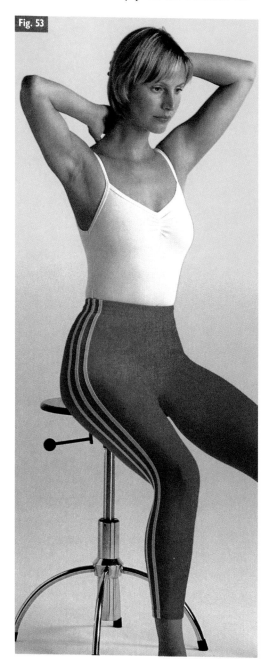

Fig. 53

tebral column into your hands. Don't raise your chin, or your will neck not be extended. Hold the contraction for 6 to 10 seconds before relaxing. Repeat four to six times.

- This exercise is even more effective with contraction-relaxation stretching. Forcefully press the back of your neck into your hands. This contracts your neck muscles isometrically. Hold the contraction for 6 to 10 seconds. Relax and immediately bend your head forward while tucking your chin in.

  To intensify the stretch, move one hand up to the back of your head and let the weight of your hand come into play (Figure 53). Hold the stretch for about 30 seconds. Slowly lift your head and concentrate on the feeling. Repeat the entire exercise four to six times.

Exercise 5: Relaxing and warming up the upper shoulder region

- Place the rolled up towel over your right shoulder so that one end hangs down in front of your body while the other end hangs down behind you. Take the front end in your left hand and the back end in your right hand. Alternate pulling the rolled up towel back and forth. Use this motion to massage your shoulder. Relax and concentrate on the feeling. Has the shoulder become pleasantly warm? Change sides.

  You can perform this excellent exercise for tension in the neck again and again without any major effort.

Exercise program 5

Standing or sitting. You need a small massage ball. You can purchase one at a medical supply store or at a sporting goods store.

Exercise I: Massage and warm-up
The massage ball is excellent for massaging and warming up your muscles, but it can also have an additional positive effect when used on the reflex zones in your feet. (Hold the massage ball between yours hands. Roll it between your palms in all directions (Figure 54). Alternate grabbing the ball with the right and left hand, as if you were about to knead it.
• A massage ball also works well for a foot massage, which acts on the entire body because of the reflex zones in your foot. Alternate placing the ball under your right foot and left foot; roll the entire sole of the foot over it (Figure 55). Feel free to exert

some pressure while doing this.
• Now, it's your shoulders' turn. Place the ball on your left shoulder with your right hand and roll it over the shoulder, back and forth and to each side. Massage the other shoulder the same way (Figure 56).
• Lean your head forward and hold it steady with your left hand. With your right hand, place the massage ball on the back of your neck and roll the

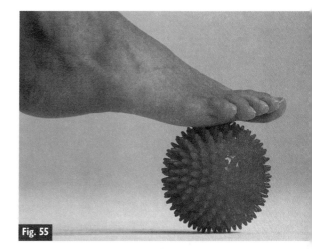

Fig. 55

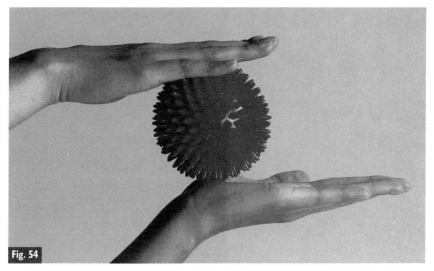

Fig. 54

ball to the right, up and down along the cervical vertebral column (Figure 57). Repeat the exercise on the other side.

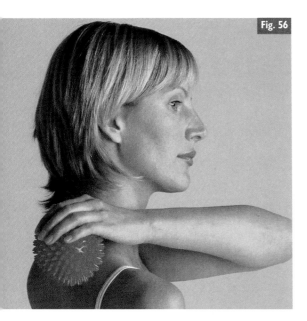

Fig. 56

Concentrate on how free your shoulders and neck have become.

Exercise 2: Relaxing the back of your head

Using the massage ball, you can give the most sensitive part of your neck, where it joins the back of your head, a good workout. In this area, the muscles have usually hardened.

• As in the last exercise, bend your head forward and place your left hand on your head. Place the ball on the uppermost point of the cervical vertebral column or in the middle of the back of the head. Massage this point with small circular motions. Initially, only exert a little pressure; later, you can increase the pressure. Switch hands now and then. Relax and concentrate on the feeling. How does the treated spot feel now?

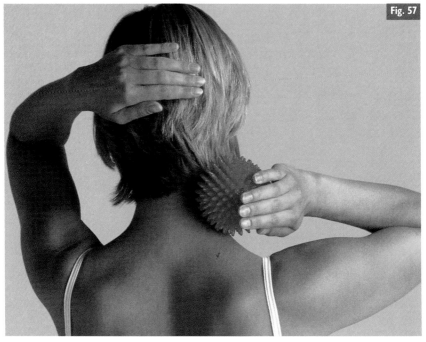

Fig. 57

Exercise 3: Mobility of the uppermost spinal column joint

The uppermost joint, where the axis and the atlas come together, is frequently jammed and blocked. The following exercise can alleviate the discomfort.

- Place your index fingers to the right and left of the back of your head. Each hand should be between the spinal column and the ear. Concentrate on the tooth of the axis. (You might want to take another look at the anatomical drawing in Figure 6 on page 11). Make very small, controlled circles with your head while you imagine how your head revolves around this "tooth." You will also feel the pressure of your fingers on the back of your head. After a while, relax your fingers, hold your head erect and relaxed, and concentrate on the feeling. How does the area feel now?

With this exercise, you should only make very small circles.

Exercise 4: Massaging the entire back of the head

Assume the same head and hand position as you did in Exercise 2. This time, however, massage the entire back of your head with the massage ball:

- Roll the ball back and forth from one ear to the other.
- Move the ball along the back of your head from your right ear to the left and back, using very small up–and–down movements.

Exercise 5: Strengthening

- Place your right hand on the right side of your neck. Press your neck against your hand without any movement (Figure 58). Allow the lateral cervical muscles to contract for 6 to 10 seconds before relaxing. Switch sides, working both sides four times each.

Exercise 6: Breathing and posture

- Extend the top of your head toward the ceiling while pulling your shoulders down. Inhale while you do this. Relax your head a little (but not completely) and lower it while moving your chin toward your sternum. Exhale during this motion. However, do not pull your shoulders forward. Your back should remain straight, and your shoulders should not change position.

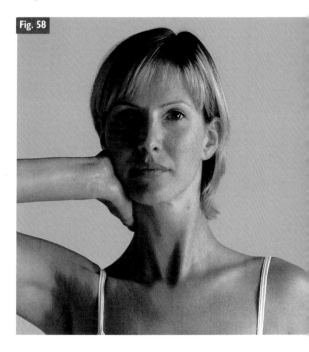

Fig. 58

Exercise program 6

Standing or sitting. You will need a towel for this exercise program.

Exercise one: Stretching
• Be sure to maintain a straight, upright posture. Tilt your head to the right as far as you can so that your right ear approaches your right shoulder. Keep your eyes focused straight ahead.

You will feel a distinct stretching in the left side of your neck. Hold the stretch for 10 to 30 seconds before you relax.

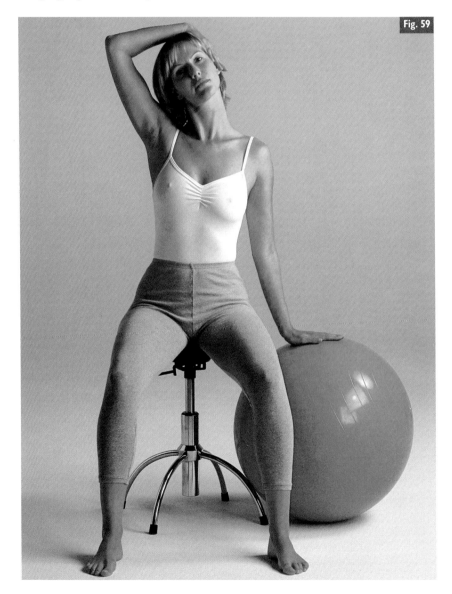

Fig. 59

- If you want to intensify the stretching, place your right hand above your head, over your left ear. However, don't pull your head down. Simply let the weight of your hand act on the side of your head. In addition, press down on your left hand with your palm facing the floor, as if you wanted to compress a large ball (Figure 59). Hold the stretch for 10 to 30 seconds. Relax and concentrate on the feeling. How does the stretched side feel? How about the other side? Change sides. Exercise each side two to four times.

- The same exercise as contraction-relaxation stretching: Assume the same head, arm, and hand position as above. First, press your head against your right hand resting on the left side of your head for about 6 seconds. Release the tension without moving your head. Gently pull your head down to the side and hold the stretch as above.

Exercise 2: Breathing

- Stand in front of a stool or chair and place your right foot on the seat of the chair. Take the rolled up towel in both hands. Bring it up above your head (Figure 60) and then to the left side.

  Bend your upper body to the left, including your head, so that your left ear approaches your left shoulder. Inhale. Notice how the air flows to the stretch. Return to the starting position, place the towel on your thigh in a relaxed manner, and slowly exhale (Figure 61). Your shoulders, muscles, and joints are now

completely relaxed. Perform the exercise four times before you change sides.

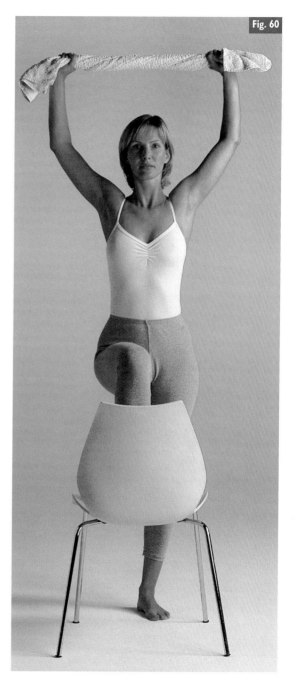

Fig. 60

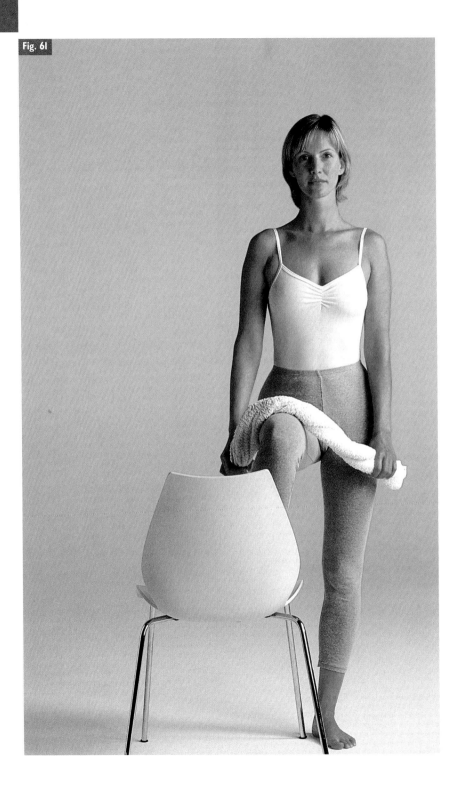

Fig. 61

Exercise 3: Stretching the chest muscles

If your chest muscles are shortened, they produce too strong a convexity in the thoracic vertebral column, exacerbating the concavity of the cervical vertebral column. For this reason, you should stretch your chest muscles regularly.

- Start by standing in front of a chair and positioning your right leg as you did in the previous exercise. Grasp the rolled up towel, pull it tight, and raise it above your head. Bend your elbows and pull the towel down behind your head (Figure 62). While contracting your abdominal and pelvic muscles to stabilize your pelvis, push the towel back away from your body. Don't pull your shoulders up!

Hold this stretch for about 30 seconds while continuing to breath normally. Relax. Repeat four times.

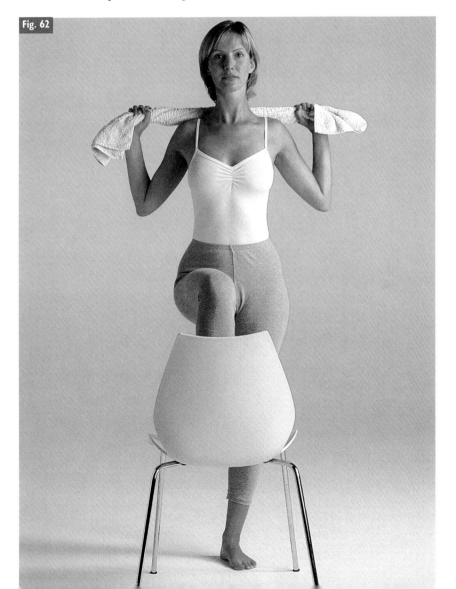

Fig. 62

Exercise 4: Strengthening and increasing mobility

- Strengthening: Place a rolled up towel on the back of your head (preferably on the lower half, just above the hairline). Hold the ends of the towel firmly. Press the back of your head against the towel and maintain the tension for 6 to 10 seconds (Figure 63). Relax briefly, but maintain the arm and towel positions. Press your head against the towel to the right for 6 to 10 seconds. Relax again. Press to the left, relax, and shake your arms and hands thoroughly. If this exercise places too much tension on your arms or shoulders, bring your arms down

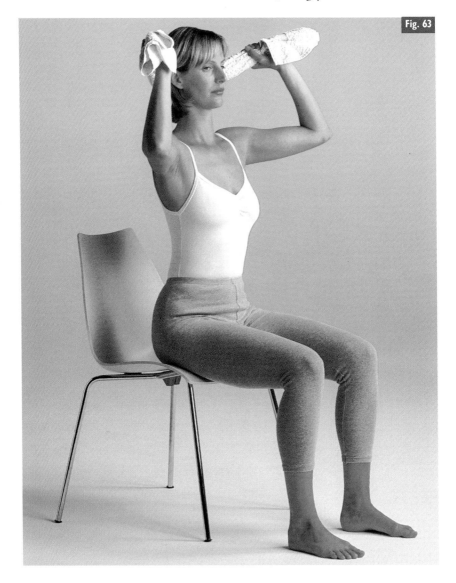

Fig. 63

briefly during each relaxation phase.

- Increasing mobility: Using the same towel position, pull the right end of the towel forward with your right hand and let your head move to the left on its own (Figure 64).

At the same time, press your chin back a little so that your neck is stretched and your head joints are more relaxed. Remain in the end position for 10 to 30 seconds before slowly returning your head to the starting position. Relax and concentrate on the feeling; then switch sides (Figure 65). Work each side three to four times.

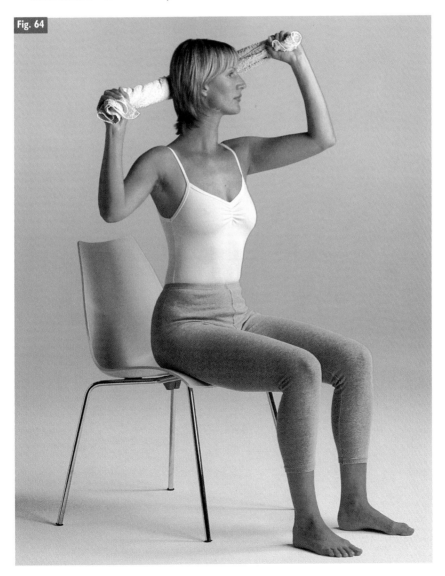

Fig. 64

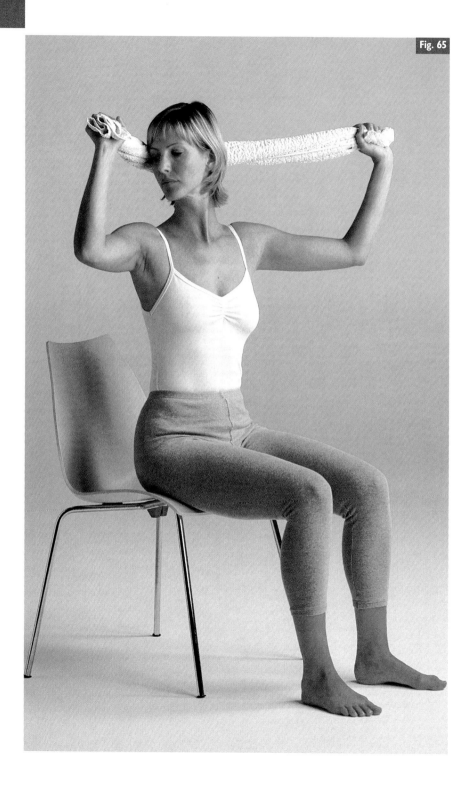

Fig. 65

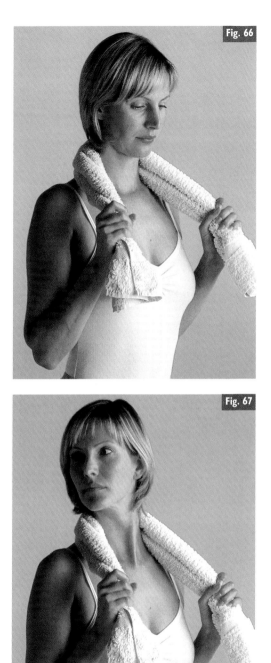

Fig. 66

Exercise 5: Increasing mobility combined with strengthening

- Place the towel around the back of your neck and grip the ends firmly. Lower your head and tuck your chin in toward your sternum; let your eyes follow the movement (Figure 66).

  Turn your head to the right (while keeping the cervical vertebral column bent) and look up to the ceiling from the corners of your eyes (Figure 67). In the end position, press your cervical vertebral column against the right part of the towel for 6 to 10 seconds. Relax and slowly return your head to the starting position. Change sides (Figure 68); work each side four times.

Fig. 67

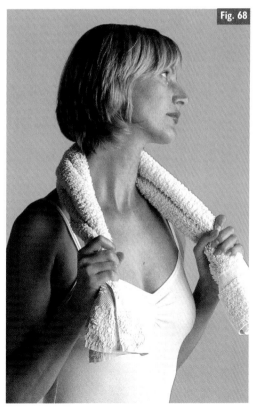

Fig. 68

Exercise program 7

Standing, resting on your hands and knees, resting on your fore-arms, and lying on your back. You will need a tennis ball and a chair with a back.

As always, start by warming up your arms and shoulders. At the same time, move your feet by jumping up and down across the room, preferably to music. Stand in front of a chair that has a high back and place your hands on the back of the chair.

Exercise I: Stretching and increasing mobility

- With your hands on the back of the chair, bend your upper body forward so that your back is straight and forms a line with your arms. Bend your knees slightly.

  Position your head between your arms with your forehead pointed down. Your eyes should be looking down at the floor (Figure 69).

  Feel the stretching in your shoulder and chest. You may also notice it in the your thighs. Turn

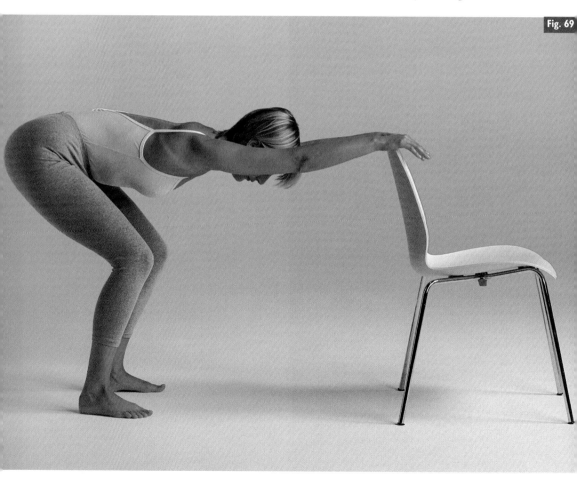

Fig. 69

your chin toward your right armpit and look in that direction. Remain in this position for 10 seconds while breathing normally. Return your head to the starting position and relax briefly. Turn your head to the left and look up to the ceiling from the corners of your eyes (Figure 70). However, don't bend your head back; it must remain between your arms. After 10 seconds, return to the starting position and switch sides (Figure 71). Work each side two to four times.

- Combine the two movements described above without returning to the starting position. Point your chin at your armpit and then turn your head to the opposite side.

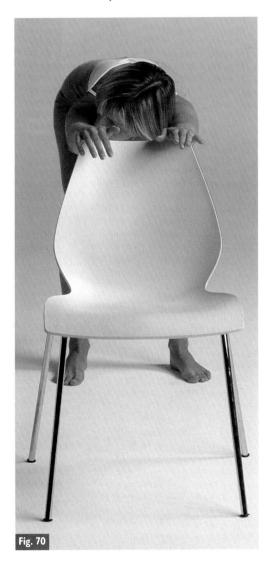

Fig. 70

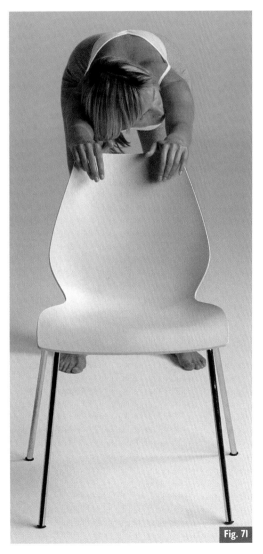

Fig. 71

Exercise 2: Strengthening

- Repeat the exercise described above on your hands and knees (Figure 72). Lower your upper body to the forearm–resting position (described below) and perform the exercise again.
- Support your weight on your knees and elbows and place your forehead on both upraised hands so that your back and neck form a line (Figure 73). Become aware of the relief and relaxation in your shoulder and neck region as well as in your cervical vertebral column. Next comes the strengthening phase. Press your forehead firmly against your hands and maintain the tension for 6 to 10 seconds before relaxing. Repeat four to six times.

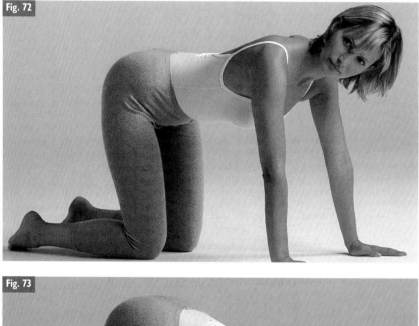

Fig. 72

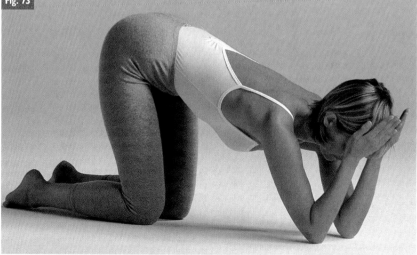

Fig. 73

Exercise 3: Mobility and awareness

- Assume the forearm-resting position once more. Your forearms should be resting on the floor about shoulder-width apart. Below your shoulder joint, your upper arms remain perpendicular to the floor.

  Place a tennis ball under your forehead and rest your forehead on it (Figure 74). You can take as much time for this resting exercise as you want.
- Roll your forehead over the ball while moving your chin toward your sternum. This extends your neck (Figure 75). Roll the ball back to the starting position. Roll back and forth a few times. This action, which involves only a small movement, relaxes your upper head joint. Concentrate on this spot while executing the movement. After you have rolled your forehead and frontal bone back and forth over the ball a few times, set the ball aside and let your forehead rest on your hands on the floor. Concentrate on relaxing for as long as you want.

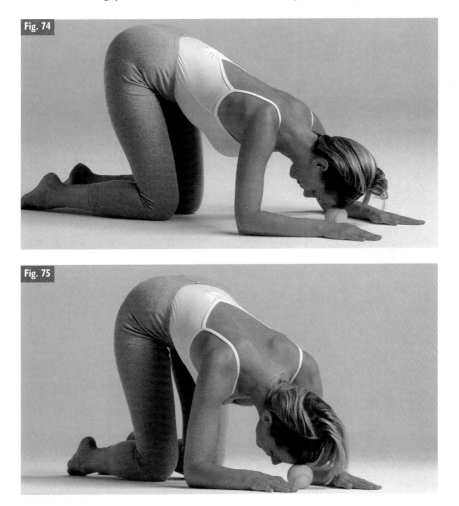

Fig. 74

Fig. 75

Exercise 4: Breathing and relaxing

This exercise will be very good for you unless the tension in your neck is especially intense. You should only remain in this exercise position for as long as you feel comfortable. With time, you will be able to hold it longer and longer.

- On your back, bend both legs at the knees or place your lower legs on a stool or other seat. Push the tennis ball under the back of your head, specifically between your ears or somewhat higher. The tip of your nose should point to the ceiling or somewhat further forward. (Be sure that it doesn't point backward because that will hyperextend your head.) Place your hands on your abdomen or at your sides on the floor in a relaxed manner (Figure 76). Transfer the weight of your head to the ball and concentrate on your breathing. Inhale through your nose and imagine how the stream of air flows along your spinal column up to the back of your head, where the ball lies. Slowly exhale through your mouth in a relaxed manner and imagine that this air is transferred from the back of your head through the ball into the floor, taking with it all your tension.
- Perform the exercise as above. Push the top of your head back as you imagine your breath flowing up to the back of your head.

  Your head will move a little over the ball, and your neck will extend even further. When exhaling, let your head return to the starting position in a relaxed manner. Readjust the ball as necessary.

This is a highly effective breathing exercise which also relaxes your head and neck muscles. Stop if it becomes uncomfortable. If you have difficulty imagining the stream of air or surrendering yourself to the above-described breathing rhythm, you should devote more effort to breathing and to breathing exercises. Relaxed breathing can have an extremely positive effect on strains and pain. Being consciously aware of your breathing will help you relax both physically and psychologically. Relaxed breathing also increases your energy, your vitality, and your ability to concentrate.

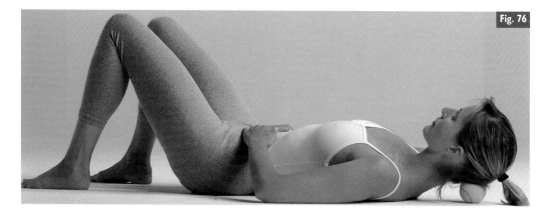

Fig. 76

Exercise program 8

Standing, sitting, and lying on your back. You'll use a small massage ball and a towel.

Exercise I: Stimulating the circulation and massaging
- Place your fingers in your hair and pull your hair up and out, ruffling it; do this over your entire head (Figures 77 and 78).

This stimulates the circulation in the area and clears the head. It works best when used only occasionally.
- Using a massage ball, you can perform another exercise that increases circulation and relaxes

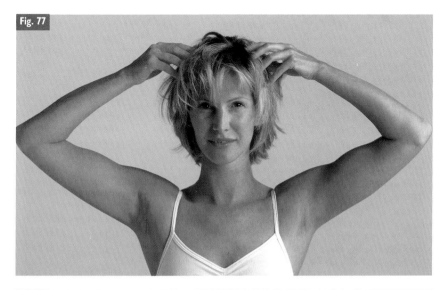

Fig. 77

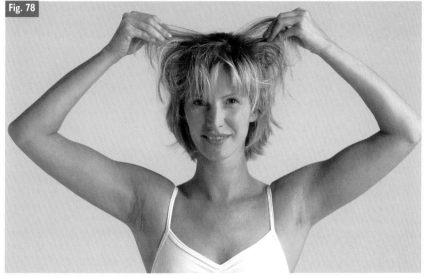

Fig. 78

the head muscles. Roll the ball over your entire head—back and forth over the back of the head, the front and top of the head, and also on the sides above the ears (Figures 79 and 80). Take the time to concentrate on the feeling. Can you feel the increased flow of blood in your scalp?

• Place the massage ball in the recess in the middle of the back of your head. Place both hands on the ball and exert pressure on it. Your elbows should point outward. Be sure that you remain loose and relaxed in the shoulder region. Maintain the tension for 6 to 10 seconds before relaxing. Repeat four to six times.

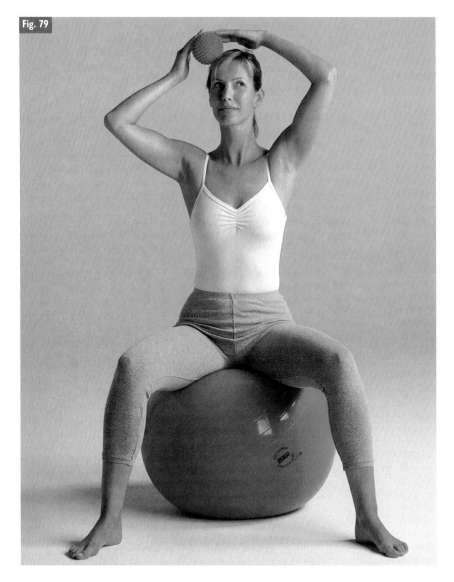

Fig. 79

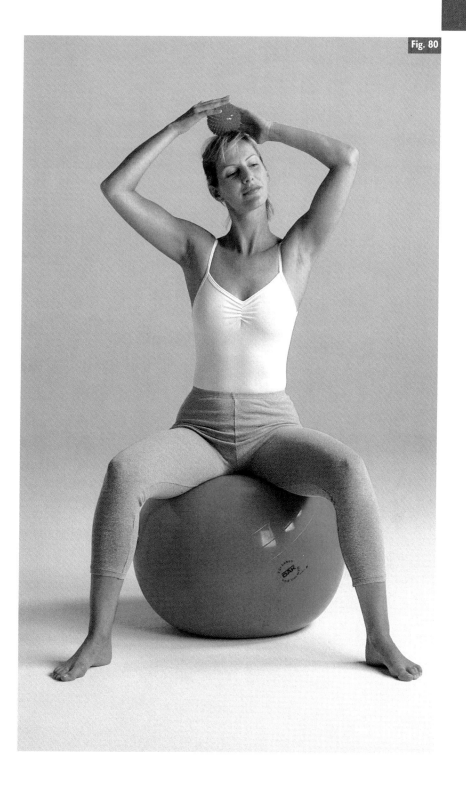

Fig. 80

Exercise 2: Strengthening

- Fold a small towel twice so that its dimensions are approximately 16 x 8 inches (40 x 20 cm). Then roll it up so that it fits in the concave area of the cervical vertebral column. Stand with your back to a wall and bend your knees slightly (or sit on a stool in front of a wall). Place the rolled up towel between your cervical vertebral column and the wall.

  Press your sacrum against the wall. Then, press your cervical vertebral column against the rolled up towel. After you have developed a feeling for the exercise, imagine wanting to push the back of your head up and to extend your neck. Hold the contraction for 6 to 10 seconds. Relax, but keep your head erect. Repeat four to six times.

- You should also strengthen your lateral cervical muscles. Place your right hand on the side of your head and press your head against your hand without moving your head (Figure 81). Maintain the tension for 6 to 10 seconds before you relax. Repeat and switch sides.

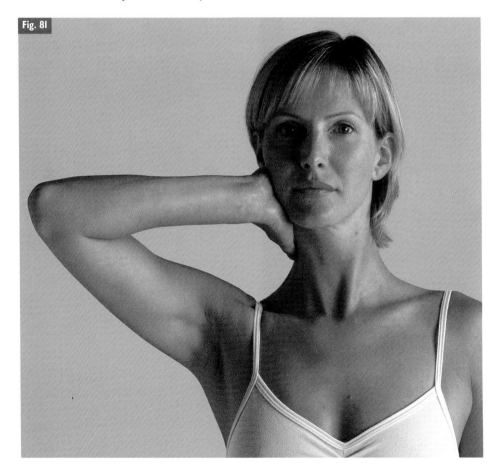

Fig. 81

Exercise 3: Increasing mobility and warming up

- Stand in front of a wall as in the previous exercise and place the massage ball in the recess in the middle of the back of your head. Press your head against the ball. Turn your head slowly over the ball to the right and left without losing momentum.

   Be sure that your chin doesn't point up. Keep it slightly taut.

   Do the exercise for as long as you want and for as long as it feels good. If the spikes on the ball bother you, you can place a towel over the ball.

Exercise 4: Strengthening

- Roll up a towel as you did in Exercise 2. Stand in a door with your right side next to the doorpost. Your right shoulder should be in front of the doorpost, touching the wall. Place the rolled up towel between the right side of your head and the doorpost and press your head against it for 6 to 10 seconds. The advantage of this exercise is that you don't have to raise your arms. Your shoulders can hang down, relaxed. Repeat the exercise four to six times on each side.

Exercise 5: Relaxing the deep neck muscles

- Lie down comfortably on your back on an exercise mat or blanket. Bend your legs at the knees or place your lower legs on a chair so that your sacrum is well-supported. Place the massage ball under your head in the recess of the back of your

head or even a little higher. Be sure you are comfortable with the position.

   If this exercise becomes uncomfortable, discontinue it by pulling the ball out and resting your head on the floor.

- Roll your head over the ball a little to the right and left. Feel the massage on the back of your head.

   Let your head rest on the ball for a moment before you pull it out. Place the back of your head on the floor and concentrate on the feeling produced by the exercise.

   How does the back of your head feel now? Do you feel the tingling and the increased circulation?

- As above, but this time, extend the top of your head back. Your head should roll over the ball a little. After 6 to 10 seconds, return to the starting position and let your head simply rest on the ball. Repeat for as long as it feels good, but don't overdo it at first.

   Pull the ball out, rest your head on the floor, and concentrate on the feeling.

> **You can also place the ball under your sacrum and put all your weight on the floor via the ball. This relaxes the pelvic-sacral region. You will feel how relaxed the area is when you pull the ball out and concentrate on your sacrum, which now lies on the floor.**

Exercise program 9

Sitting or standing and resting on the forearms. You will need a resistance band (a long rubber band made of latex). You can find this in sporting goods store in various strengths and colors. It is especially helpful for strengthening and for stretching exercises.

Exercise I: Warming up, breathing, and stretching

- While walking, standing, or sitting, grab the resistance band at about shoulder height and swing it in all possible directions, both in front of and behind your body (Figures 82 and 83).
- With the resistance band taut

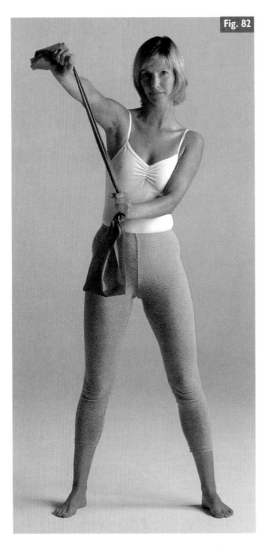

Fig. 82

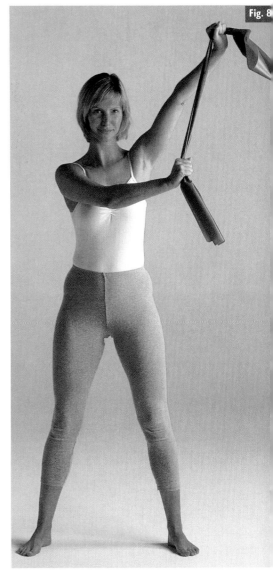

Fig. 8

between your hands, bring both arms up high above your head, inhaling as you do so (Figure 84). While bringing your arms back down and relaxing your grip on the resistance band, exhale slowly in a relaxed manner (Figure 85). Repeat two to four times.

• Place the resistance band over your right shoulder and grab it in front with your right hand and in back with your left hand at about chest height (Figure 86).

Tighten the band by pulling down on both ends and consciously let it pull your shoulder down. Extend your head upward and lean to the right so that your right ear approaches your

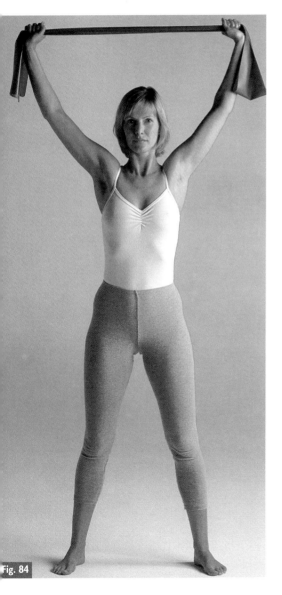

Fig. 84

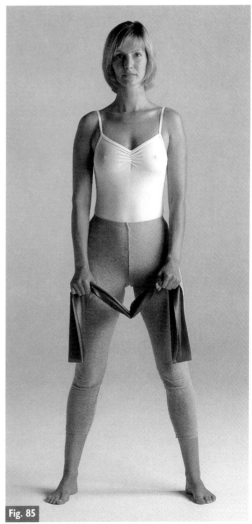

Fig. 85

right shoulder (Figure 87).

Hold the stretch for about 30 seconds. Release the tension, straighten your head, and concentrate on the feeling. Change sides. Repeat four times per side.

- The exercise has a more intense effect if you lean your head to the opposite side.

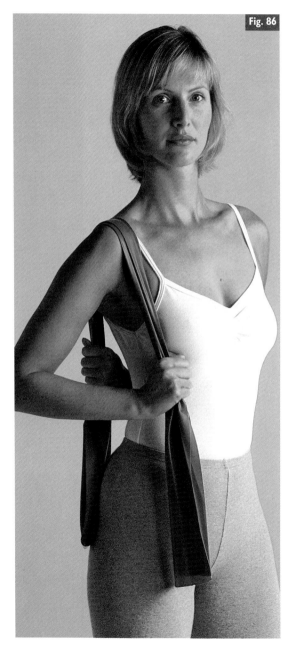

Fig. 86

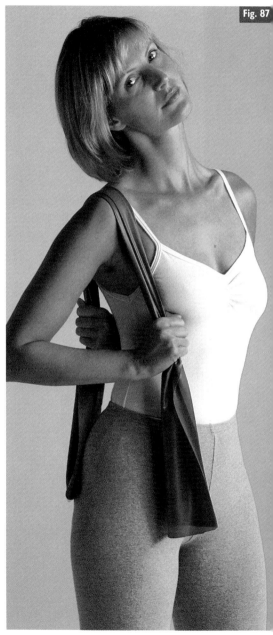

Fig. 87

Exercise 2: Strengthening

- Fold the resistance band in half and place it around the back of your neck. (If the material is uncomfortable against your skin, place a towel between your neck and the latex. This also protects the band, which should not get wet.)

Press the band against your neck for 6 to 10 seconds before you relax (Figure 88). Repeat four to six times.

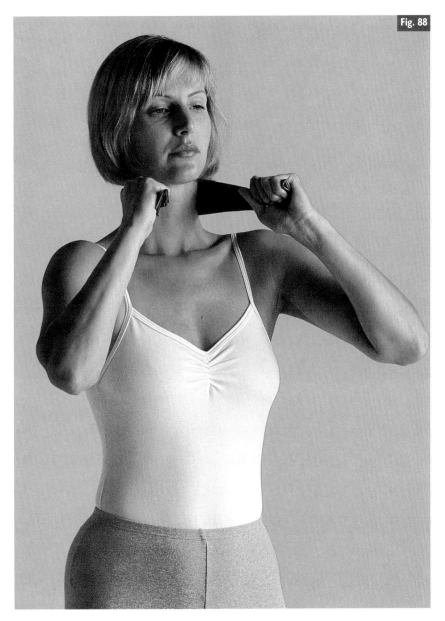

Fig. 88

Exercise 3: Stretching, warming up, and increasing mobility

- Place the resistance band on the top of the back of your head and pull it forward and down. (You might want to place a towel between your head and the band.) Bend your head forward and rotate your head to the right against the resistance of the band. Look at your right shoulder (Figure 89). Hold this end position for 6 to 10 seconds and continue to breathe normally.

Rotate your head back to the starting position and straighten it. Concentrate on the feeling for a while before changing sides (Figure 90). Repeat four times per side.

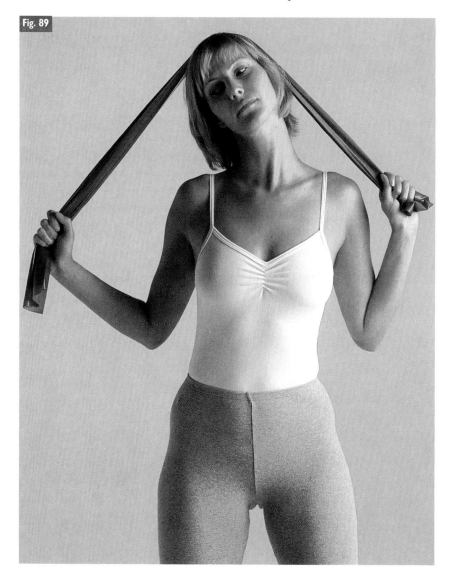

Fig. 89

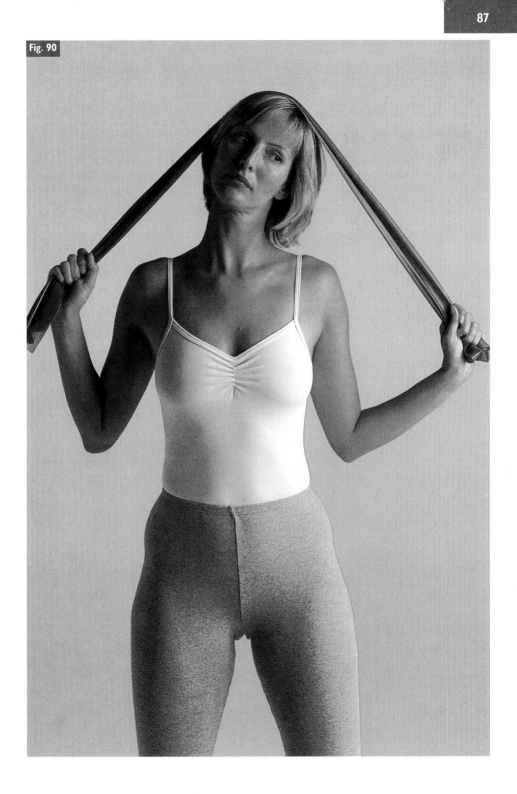

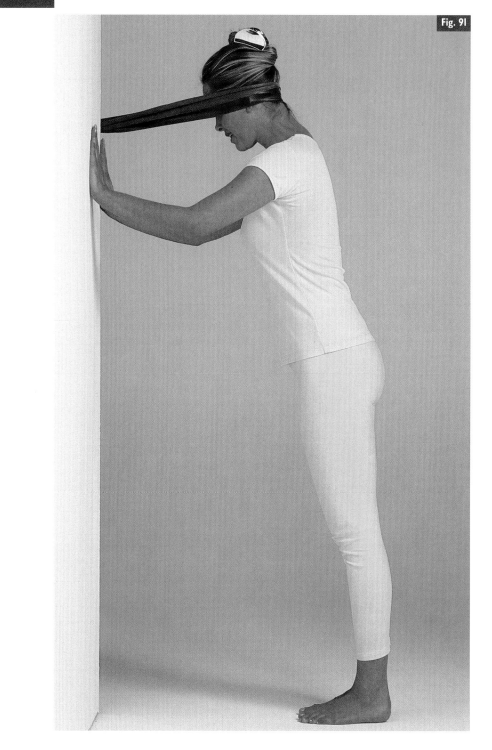

Fig. 91

Exercise 4: Strengthening

- Stand a foot or more away from a wall and hold the resistance band in both hands. The band should be somewhat longer than shoulder width. Place the band around the back of your head and lean forward with your upper body at a slight angle. Support yourself on the wall with both hands, still gripping the band. Your entire body should form a straight line with your elbows slightly bent. You can also secure the band using a door instead of your hands (Figure 91). Consciously tighten your abdominal and gluteal muscles to stabilize your pelvis and remove any concavity that isn't physiological.

  Press your head back against the resistance of the band, extending your elbows a little. However, don't lean your head back. Hold the contraction for 6 to 10 seconds before releasing the tension. Repeat the exercise four to six times.

  Relax and become aware of your erect head posture. You may now feel that you can support and balance your head more easily.

- Perform very small, minimal nodding movements with your head.

Exercise 5: Stretching and posture

- Start by tying the ends of the resistance band in a knot. Sit on the floor and pull your legs in close to your body in a crouching position. Place the resistance band under your knees and pull the other end over your head.

  You can fold a small towel and place it between the band and your head if that is more comfortable. Place your hands on your lower legs in a relaxed manner. Be sure to keep your back straight. Extend your head upward against the taut and resistant rubber band. Keep your shoulders down. You can also pull them farther down. Hold the tension for 10 or more seconds, but only for as long as you can comfortably stretch. Stop immediately if the tension becomes unpleasant.

  Remove the band from around your head, relax, and concentrate on what you are feeling. Repeat two to four times.

- Assume the same exercise position, but this time lower your head and let the taut band work on the back of your head. You should feel the stretch in the neck region. Hold for 10 to 30 seconds, but stop if it becomes uncomfortable. Relax and concentrate on the feeling.

Exercise 6: Relaxing

- Lie on the floor with the folded towel under your head. Bend your legs at the knees or place your lower legs on a stool. Inhale and exhale while completely relaxed. Feel your breathing. Can you feel it in your abdomen?

  After a while, consciously inhale and exhale from the neck. Can you feel how your neck stretches a little when inhaling and relaxes when exhaling? Concentrate on your breathing while completely still and relaxed.

  Relax even more, until all your neck muscles are free of tension. Don't forget to keep your facial muscles completely relaxed so that your entire head region is free of tension.

Stiff neck after sleeping?

We often hear patients or acquaintances say, "I woke up with a stiff neck." In most cases, the discomfort does not stop at the neck. The pain actually migrates up from the back of the head, often up to the eyes. Headaches frequently result from strained shoulder and neck muscles.

These strains may be the result of poor posture habits, perhaps at the computer or cash register, but they may also result from continuous or excessive emotional or physical stress. If the pain is noticeable primarily after getting up out of bed, a draft (cold muscles contract and increase their tension in order to generate warmth) or even an improper sleeping position may be the cause.

Where and how do you sleep?

The right mattress

To avoid back and neck problems the next morning, you should invest in a good mattress. This should be a one-piece unit that supports the body, is elastic at every point, and does not sink in under the pelvis, shoulders, or head. The mattress should support the lumbar and cervical vertebral columns.

The mattress should not give when you turn or move. The important point is that the spinal column should rest in its natural position.

The pillow

Pillows that are too soft and too large are still the commercial norm. They can cause problems. To support your neck, your head should rest on a small, hard pillow. We recommend special pillows that support the back of the neck. Some even come with a specially adjusted roll for the cervical vertebral column. The pillow should be neither too high nor too low, otherwise the pillow forces the cervical vertebral column into an improperly curved position (Figure 92). Your neck muscles tighten up, and you wake up with a stiff neck. The pillow should be high enough so that the thoracic and cervical vertebral columns are in a straight

Figure 92 Pillows must provide the correct level of support.

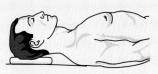

support is too low

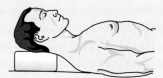

support is too high

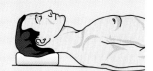

support is the correct height

line. This is true whether you are on your back, side, or stomach.

Sleeping positions

Sleeping on your stomach
We don't recommend this position. The spinal column is in an unnaturally concave position. You have to turn your neck so that your head can lie on its side. The shoulder muscles on one side can become cramped, and you wake up with a strained neck.

Sleeping on your back
This position is better, but not ideal. The lumbar vertebral column cannot relax completely. To support this portion of the spine, you should place a thick pillow under your knees. This position is acceptable for the head and neck region if the pillow is the correct height.

Sleeping on your side
Sleeping on your side with your knees slightly bent (the fetal position) is the best position for your back (Figure 93).

Your shoulder is not on the pillow, but in front of it. This maintains the natural (straight) line between your neck and the thoracic vertebral regions.

Pulling your knees up relieves the tension on the lumbar vertebral column. A pillow between the knees is also helpful.

Exercises for a tense neck

If you wake up in the morning with a stiff neck, or if you feel tense during the day and want to take a break, choose one or more of the brief, effective exercises from the following list.

- Roll up a towel along its length. Heat it up by placing it on a heater or in the oven for a few minutes or by dipping it briefly in hot water. Place it on the back of the neck and let the warmth spread.

  You can also hold the towel near its ends and alternate pulling it forward to the right and left, massaging your neck and cramped muscles (Figure 94).

- Using the fingers of both hands,

Figure 93
In the ideal sleep position, the spinal column is in its natural position, the head lies at the correct level, the cervical vertebral column has support, and the mattress adjusts to the body's shape.

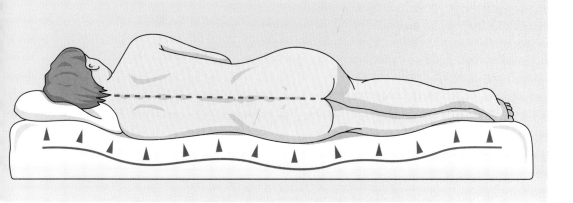

massage your neck to the right and left of the spinal column from top to bottom. If you like, you may continue out to the shoulders.

- Pull your shoulders all the way up to your ears and let them drop back heavily. Repeat ten to twenty times.
- Roll your shoulders in circles. Roll forward a few times, then backward a few times. Alternate between making large and small circles.
- Stand against a wall, place a book on your head, and try to push it toward the ceiling. At the same time, slide your fingertips far down along your legs. You should perform this exercise several times a day because it extends shortened neck muscles and relieves the neck of tension. Relax frequently during the exercise.
- Use a small massage ball to massage away your pain. Stand about 12 inches (30 cm) from a wall. Lean your back against the wall and place the ball at about ear level between the back of your head and the wall.

    Press your head back against the ball; then, turn your head slightly to the right and left. This will massage away the tension in the small muscles in your neck.
- Place the massage ball on one shoulder. Using the opposite hand, massage the hard shoulder muscles with the ball.
- Try this effective exercise to relieve strains in your neck. Lean your head to the right side so that your right ear approaches your right shoulder. Place

your right hand on the left side of your head so that your fingertips are almost on your ear. While holding the head in this position (do not pull or bounce), reach toward the floor with your left hand. Hold the stretch for 10 to 30 seconds while continuing to breathe normally. Repeat three times on each side.

Afterward, you will no doubt feel some relief.

- Fold both hands and place them on the back of your head. Press your head forcefully against your hands.

    After 8 to 10 seconds, release the tension briefly. Repeat four to six times. Bend your head forward and let the weight of your hands come into play. Continue to breathe normally. Hold the stretch for 20 to 30 seconds.
- Rotate your head to your right and lower your chin to your shoulder. Rotate your head 180° to your left shoulder so that your chin describes a semicircle. Move your head back and forth between your shoulders several times.

Strained neck muscles are often associated with strained head and facial muscles and vice versa. Therefore, you should also loosen up the latter muscles by massaging them with your fingers and by relaxing.

Acupressure points for the neck and shoulders

Pressing special acupressure points can stimulate the flow of energy to tense regions of the body. Such a treatment, especially in the neck-cranial base region can relieve tension and restore circulation that is frequently impaired. The advantage of acupressure, as opposed to acupuncture, is that you can perform it yourself. You can use acupressure, also called pressure point massage, on all areas. It relieves

Fig. 94

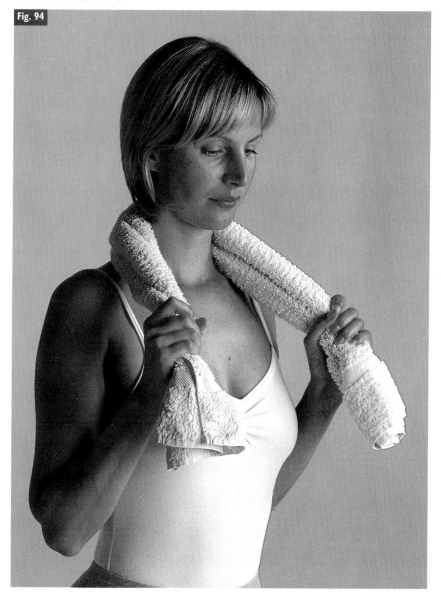

morning neck pain and stimulates the circulation in the head region. Thus, it is beneficial for headaches, fatigue symptoms, and lack of concentration.

Performing acupressure

> **Rule of thumb: You should clearly feel the pressure but not any actual pain.**

Because many points are located symmetrically on both sides of the body, you use acupressure simultaneously on your right and left side. Press each point for about 30 seconds, but feel free to continue to hold the pressure for as long as it is comfortable.

Important pressure points in the back of the neck

- Place the finger pads of both your middle or index fingers on the acupressure points. Press on the points in order, that is, from the middle of the cranial base along the bone to the outside, then right and left along the cervical vertebrae (Figure 95).
- Alternately, you can move through the circuit with varying pressure. Your thumbs are also well-suited for the points along the cranial base. In this case, apply your fingers on the back of your head.
- You'll find another important acupressure point exactly between the seventh cervical vertebra and the external edge of the shoulder. This point helps

relieve tension in the shoulders and neck. All three fingerpads can exert pressure on this point, simultaneously or with your right hand on your left shoulder and vice versa.
- Finally, stick all your fingers in your hair and let the finger pads rest on your scalp. Press on these points and gently circle them. Move your fingers and press the scalp again. This way, you can treat the entire scalp. Afterward, your head will feel light and relaxed.

Tips for your everyday routine

By using simple preventive measures in your everyday activities, you can avoid having a stiff neck or tension in the region of the cervical vertebral column:

- Be sure to maintain an erect posture throughout your everyday routine. If at all possible, your head should rarely be bent too far, especially too far backward.
- Support your head when reading, driving, or working with your hands. In addition, you should always schedule sufficient breaks.
- Support the book when you are reading.
- Use an inclined lectern placed on top of your desk when you are writing.
- Place the computer monitor at eye level or somewhat lower, just the way you would place a television screen.
- Adjust the handlebars of your

bicycle so that they are high enough that you can keep the entire spinal column straight, including the neck.

- Keep your eyes forward when walking or running. Don't pull your chin up; tuck it in slightly.
- Don't hold your head high when swimming the breast-stroke. This position can injure the cervical vertebral column. Therefore, use the backstroke or keep your head in the water with the breaststroke.
- Avoid rotating your head abruptly.
- Do not expose the back of your neck to drafts.
- Avoid working above head level; use a stepladder.
- Avoid sitting in the front row in the theater, movies, or lecture hall.
- Train your neck muscles and the other retaining muscles daily.

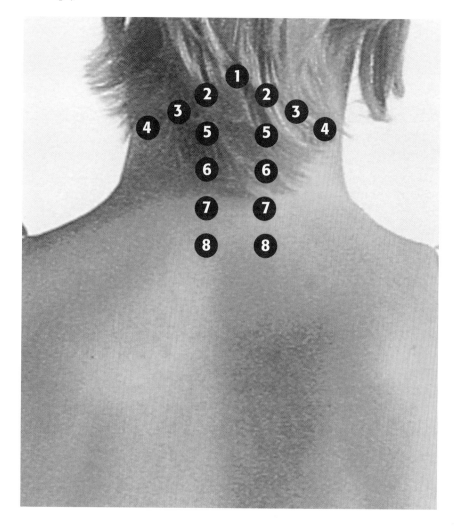

Index